Anterior Segment

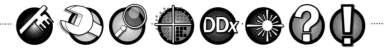

Rapid Diagnosis in Ophthalmology
Series Editors: Jay S. Duker MD, Marian S. Macsai MD
Associate Editor: Gary S. Schwartz MD

Anterior Segment
Bruno Machado Fontes, Marian S. Macsai
ISBN 978-0-323-04406-6

Lens and Glaucoma
Joel S. Schuman, Viki Christopoulos, Deepinder K. Dhaliwal,
Malik Y. Kahook, Robert J. Noecker
ISBN 978-0-323-04443-1

Neuro-ophthalmology
Jonathan D. Trobe
ISBN 978-0-323-04456-1

Oculoplastic and Reconstructive Surgery
Jeffrey A. Nerad, Keith D. Carter, Mark Alford
ISBN 978-0-323-05386-0

Pediatric Ophthalmology and Strabismus
Mitchell B. Strominger
ISBN 978-0-323-05168-2

Retina
Adam H. Rogers, Jay S. Duker
ISBN 978-0-323-04959-7

Commissioning Editor: Russell Gabbedy
Development Editor: Martin Mellor Publishing Services Ltd
Project Manager: Rory MacDonald
Design Manager: Stewart Larking
Illustration Manager: Merlyn Harvey
Illustrator: Jennifer Rose
Marketing Manager(s) (UK/USA): John Canelon/Lisa Damico

Series Editors: Jay S. **Duker** MD, Marian S. **Macsai** MD

Associate Editor: Gary S. **Schwartz** MD

Rapid Diagnosis in Ophthalmology
Anterior
Segment

By
Marian S. Macsai MD
Chief, Division of Ophthalmology, Evanston Northwestern Healthcare;
Professor and Vice-Chair, Department of Ophthalmology, Feinberg
School of Medicine, Northwestern University, Chicago, IL, USA

Bruno Machado Fontes MD
Cornea and Refractive Surgery Fellow, Feinberg School of Medicine,
Northwestern University, Chicago, IL, USA; Evanston Northwestern
Healthcare, Evanston, IL, USA; Federal University of Sao Paulo, Brazil

Series Editors
Jay S. Duker MD
Director, New England Eye Center, Vitreoretinal Diseases and Surgery
Service; Professor and Chair of Ophthalmology, Tufts University School
of Medicine, Boston, MA, USA

Marian S. Macsai MD
Chief, Division of Ophthalmology, Evanston Northwestern Healthcare;
Professor and Vice-Chair, Department of Ophthalmology, Feinberg
School of Medicine, Northwestern University, Chicago, IL, USA

Associate Editor
Gary S. Schwartz MD
Adjunct Associate Professor, Department of Ophthalmology,
University of Minnesota, Minneapolis, MN, USA

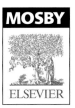

MOSBY

ELSEVIER

Mosby is an affiliate of Elsevier Inc.

First published 2008

ISBN 978-0-323-04406-6

British Library Cataloguing in Publication Data
A catalogue record for this book is available from the British Library

Library of Congress Cataloging in Publication Data
A catalog record for this book is available from the Library of Congress

Notice
Medical knowledge is constantly changing. Standard safety precautions must be followed, but as new research and clinical experience broaden our knowledge, changes in treatment and drug therapy may become necessary or appropriate. Readers are advised to check the most current product information provided by the manufacturer of each drug to be administered to verify the recommended dose, the method and duration of administration, and contraindications. It is the responsibility of the practitioner, relying on experience and knowledge of the patient, to determine dosages and the best treatment for each individual patient. Neither the Publisher nor the authors assume any liability for any injury and/or damage to persons or property arising from this publication.

The Publisher

your source for books,
journals and multimedia
in the health sciences
www.elsevierhealth.com

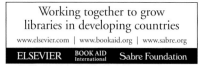

Working together to grow
libraries in developing countries
www.elsevier.com | www.bookaid.org | www.sabre.org

ELSEVIER   BOOK AID International   Sabre Foundation

The publisher's policy is to use **paper manufactured from sustainable forests**

Printed in China
Last digit is the print number: 9 8 7 6 5 4 3 2 1

Contents

Contents

Given the complexity and quantity of clinical knowledge required to correctly identify and treat ocular disease, a quick reference text with high quality color images represents an invaluable resource to the busy clinician. Despite the availability of extensive resources online to clinicians, accessing these resources can be time consuming and often requires filtering through unnecessary information. In the exam room, facing a patient with an unfamiliar presentation or complicated medical problem, this series will be an invaluable resource.

This handy pocket sized reference series puts the knowledge of world-renowned experts at your fingertips. The standardized format provides the key element of each disease entity as your first encounter. The additional information on the clinical presentation, ancillary testing, differential diagnosis and treatment, including the prognosis, allows the clinician to instantly diagnose and treat the most common diseases seen in a busy practice. Inclusion of classical clinical color photos provides additional assurance in securing an accurate diagnosis and initiating management.

Regardless of the area of the world in which the clinician practices, these handy references guides will provide the necessary resources to both diagnose and treat a wide variety of ophthalmic diseases in all ophthalmologic specialties. The clinician who does not have easy access to sub-specialists in Anterior Segment, Glaucoma, Pediatric Ophthalmology, Strabismus, Neuro-ophthalmology, Retina, Oculoplastic and Reconstructive Surgery, and Uveitis will find these texts provide an excellent substitute. World-wide recognized experts equip the clinician with the elements needed to accurately diagnose treat and manage these complicated diseases, with confidence aided by the excellent color photos and knowledge of the prognosis.

The field of knowledge continues to expand for both the clinician in training and in practice. As a result we find it a challenge to stay up to date in the diagnosis and management of every disease entity that we face in a busy clinical practice. This series is written by an international group of experts who provide a clear, structured format with excellent photos.

It is our hope that with the aid of these six volumes, the clinician will be better equipped to diagnose and treat the diseases that affect their patients, and improve their lives.

Marian S. Macsai and Jay S. Duker

Preface

We face challenging cases in practice every day, and often textbooks are not at hand. Searching the internet, when available, may yield information that is not always reliable. In anterior segment diseases signs and symptoms can overlap, and minor details will differentiate them. Trustworthy, easy to use, light-weight, illustrated books can be extremely helpful, especially when the prognosis of a specific disease depends on rapid diagnosis and initiation of the correct treatment.

The main goal of this book is to provide the most important features of anterior segment pathologies, for use as a quick-reference tool in daily practice. In addition to a diagnostic and treatment guide, we discuss the prognosis of each specific disease entity. High quality photos are displayed alongside every condition, so the practitioner can more easily establish the correct diagnosis for each patient. The standard chapter algorithm (key aspects, clinical findings, ancillary testing, differential diagnosis, treatment and prognosis) was created so it can be reliably used as a structured diagnostic and therapeutic plan.

Several sources were accessed, and information was compressed in every chapter. Words were carefully chosen to be meaningful and help the practitioner make a rapid and precise diagnosis of a number of anterior segment pathologies. We hope that this book will be a useful and powerful resource for ocular health professionals all over the world.

Bruno M. Fontes, MD
Marian S. Macsai, MD

To my beloved wife Tatiana, my family, friends and contributors. Thanks very much for your support.

Bruno Machado Fontes

Dedication

Section 1

Developmental Anomalies of the Anterior Segment

Axenfeld–Rieger Syndrome

Key Facts

- Autosomal dominant with high penetrance
- Developmental anterior segment abnormalities secondary to abnormal migration of neural crest cells
- Almost always bilateral
- High incidence of secondary glaucoma (≥50% risk)
- No sex predilection
- **Three genetic loci identified:** chromosomes 4q25, 6p25, and 13q14

Clinical Findings

- Posterior embryotoxon (prominent and anteriorly displaced Schwalbe's line)
- Iris stromal hypoplasia, abnormalities of pupil shape (corectopia), number (polycoria), and sometimes persistent papillary membrane
- **Other ocular abnormalities include:**
  - iris coloboma • sclerocornea • limbal dermoids • strabismus • retinal degenerations • microphthalmos
- **Most common systemic associations:**
  - facial (maxillary hypoplasia, telecanthus, hypertelorism, broad and flat nasal bridge) • dental (anodontia, hypodontia, microdontia) • umbilical (redundant periumbilical skin)

Ancillary Testing

- Assess family history—examine family members
- Gonioscopy
- Optic nerve examination for glaucomatous damage
- Refer to a pediatrician—systemic associations often present

Differential Diagnosis

- Iridocorneal endothelial syndromes • Iridoschisis

Treatment

- **Glaucoma control:**
  - primarily with topical medications • may require surgery—trabeculectomy is often the first choice, followed by tube shunts if the former fails (laser trabeculoplasty is not a good option because of angle abnormality)

Prognosis

- Good if no other ocular abnormality associated and good glaucoma control
- Iris abnormalities usually stationary

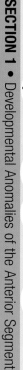

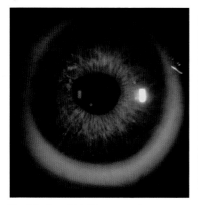

Fig. 1.1 Axenfeld–Rieger syndrome: corectopia, posterior embryotoxon, and generalized iris hypoplasia.

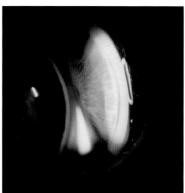

Fig. 1.2 Gonioscopy showing pronounced iris processes extending across the angle and inserting into Schwalbe's line.

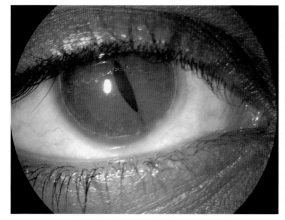

Fig. 1.3 Axenfeld syndrome: a 9-year-old girl with corectopia, prominent Schwalbe's line, and anterior synechiae. Her glaucoma was controlled with topical timolol and dorzolamide. She had best corrected vision of 20/200 in both eyes and no systemic abnormalities. (Courtesy of Ruiz S. Alonso, MD.)

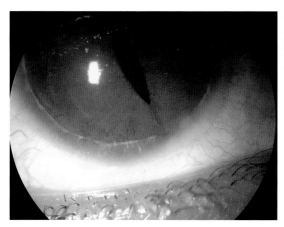

Fig. 1.4 A more detailed image of the patient in Fig. 1.3. (Courtesy of Ruiz S. Alonso, MD.)

Peters Anomaly

Key Facts

- Phenotypically heterogeneous condition associated with multiple underlying ocular (mostly anterior segment) and systemic defects
- Sporadic (most common), autosomal dominant, and autosomal recessive forms described
- Bilateral in 60–80% of cases
- High risk of early onset glaucoma

Clinical Findings

- Characterized by central corneal opacification secondary to a posterior corneal defect (absence or marked attenuation of the endothelium and Descemet's membrane)
- Corneal adhesion to the lens and/or iris
- Density of corneal defect is variable; histopathologically, there are abnormalities at all layers
- Corneal neovascularization is uncommon
- **Systemic abnormalities include:**
  - developmental delay • congenital heart disease • external ear abnormalities • structural defects of the central nervous system • genitourinary malformations • cleft lip or palate • hearing loss and spinal defects

Ancillary Testing

- Ocular ultrasonography (A and B scan)
- Ultrasound biomicroscopy
- Examinations under anesthesia usually required

Differential Diagnosis

- Primary congenital glaucoma
- Congenital hereditary endothelial dystrophy
- Birth trauma
- Mucopolysaccharidoses

Treatment

- Surgical (keratoplasty)—typically complex and challenging
- May require lensectomy, anterior segment reconstruction
- In unilateral cases, intensive amblyopia treatment required to achieve best outcomes
- Genetic evaluation

Prognosis

- Often associated with a poor visual outcome
- Long-term graft clarity achieved in only 36% of eyes (mostly first grafts)
- Surgical intervention involving one or more procedures is effective in controlling IOP in 32% of eyes with associated congenital glaucoma
  - Still, multiple procedures and adjunctive medical therapy are often required to achieve and maintain adequate IOP control

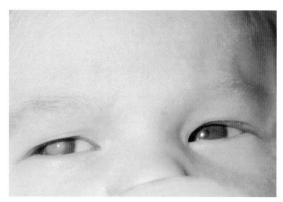

Fig. 1.5 Peters anomaly: a baby with unilateral involvement. Note central corneal opacity.

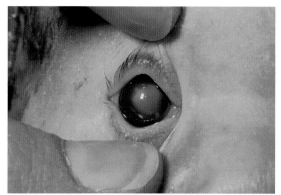

Fig. 1.6 A more detailed image of the patient in Fig. 1.5. The corneal periphery is clear.

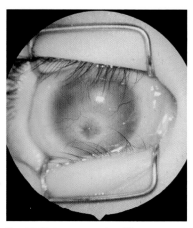

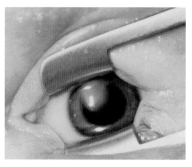

Fig. 1.7 Peters anomaly: diffuse corneal edema with neovascularization, lipid deposition, and an area of ulceration. This patient had Descemet's membrane and endothelium absence, as well as anterior adherence of iris and lens.

Fig. 1.8 Localized involvement in a child with Peters anomaly.

Aniridia

Key Facts

- Most common cause of congenital limbal stem cell deficiency
- Bilateral—can occur as a sporadic isolated condition or in association with Wilms tumor, genitourinary abnormalities, and mental retardation (WAGR) syndrome
- Family members may have variable presentations, with clinical aniridia in some and others with atypical iris defects ranging from radial clefts to atypical colobomas
- Chromosomal aberrations are frequent
- **Associated with:**
  - glaucoma • foveal and optic nerve hypoplasia • nystagmus • progressive keratopathy • cataract

Clinical Findings

- Iris findings range from clinically normal to focal or total absence of pupillary rim
- Often no visible central iris tissue
- A stump of iris tissue peripherally is present in nearly all cases (gonioscopy sometimes needed to visualize)
- **Keratopathy:**
  - starts as thickened and irregular peripheral epithelium with neovascularization
  - will extend centrally throughout patient's lifetime
  - chronic epitheliopathy will lead to subepithelial fibrosis and stromal scarring

Ancillary Testing

- Ultrasound biomicroscopy (assess anterior segment anatomy, when corneal scarring limits view)
- A scan (assess posterior segment, control and evaluate glaucoma treatment efficacy in children)
- Impression cytology to evaluate stem cell deficiency
- Optical coherence tomography to confirm foveal hypoplasia if media clear
- Examine family members
- MRI to look for Wilms tumor

Differential Diagnosis

- Peters anomaly
- Congenital glaucoma (can be associated)
- Axenfeld–Rieger syndrome

Treatment

- Refer to geneticist and pediatrician to evaluate possible genetic and systemic abnormalities
- Treat dry eye state aggressively (lubricants, bandage contact lens, tarsorrhaphy)
- Glaucoma control (surgical intervention often required)
- Amblyopia treatment
- Penetrating or lamellar keratoplasty associated with limbal stem cell transplantation

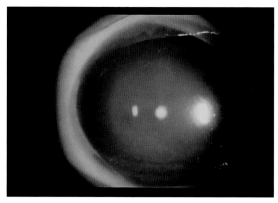

Fig. 1.9 Aniridia. Note diffuse corneal loss of luster and opacity associated with stem cell deficiency and glaucoma.

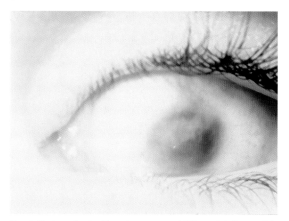

Fig. 1.10 A patient with sclerocornea (differential diagnosis): undistinct corneal margins, opacity, and neovascularization. This can rarely be associated with aniridia.

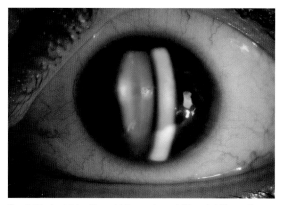

Fig. 1.11 A child with aniridia, cataract (Fig. 1.12), and congenital glaucoma. (Courtesy of Mario M. Araujo, MD.)

Aniridia (Continued)

Prognosis

- Degree of foveal hypoplasia is the strongest determining factor of visual potential in children
- Cataract, aniridic keratopathy (with painful recurrent corneal ulcerations), and glaucoma are common complications as patients age
- Blindness occurs frequently
- Because the keratopathy is secondary to abnormal limbal stem cells, traditional penetrating keratopathy will fail without adjunctive limbal stem cell transplantation

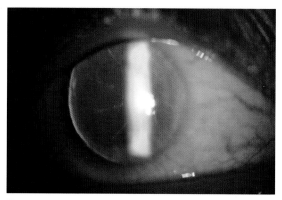

Fig. 1.12 Associated cataract in the same patient as in Fig. 1.11. (Courtesy of Mario M. Araujo, MD.)

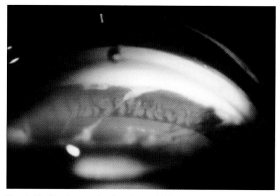

Fig. 1.13 Gonioscopic view in a child with aniridia. Note ciliary process and iris strands. (Courtesy of Guilherme Rocha, MD.)

Section 2

Disorders of the Tear Film

Aqueous Deficiency

Key Facts

- Reduced tear production associated with symptoms of ocular discomfort
- More frequent in elderly patients and women (hormone related in most cases)
- **Symptoms include:**
  - dry sensation • irritation • tearing • burning • stinging • foreign body sensation • photophobia • blurry vision • redness • mucous discharge • increased frequency of blinking

Clinical Findings

- Thin or discontinuous tear meniscus
- Increased debris and unstable tear film
- Delayed tear clearance

Ancillary Testing

- Tear break-up time
- Schirmer testing
- Ocular surface dye staining (fluorescein, rose bengal or lissamine green)
- Impression cytology

Differential Diagnosis

- Meibomian gland disease
- Blink or lid abnormality
- Exposure or neurotrophic keratopathy

Treatment

- Elimination of exacerbating exogenous factors
- Topical lubrication (artificial tears and ointments) or autologous serum
- Topical cyclosporin A
- Punctal occlusion
- Investigate secondary causes (e.g. Sjögren syndrome, HIV infection, vitamin A deficiency)

Prognosis

- Heterogenous condition in severity, duration, and etiology
- Usually not curable and the chronicity may lead to patient frustration
- Initially not sight-threatening and is characterized by troublesome, non-severe symptoms of irritation
- Reversible conjunctival squamous metaplasia and punctate epithelial erosions of the conjunctiva and cornea may develop in moderate to severe cases
  - Patients with severe aqueous deficiency can develop complications such as ocular surface keratinization or corneal ulceration, scarring, thinning, or neovascularization

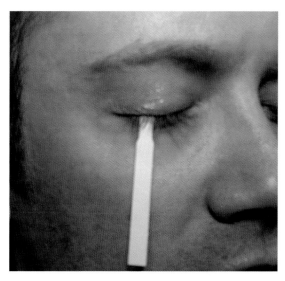

Fig. 2.1 Schirmer test: strip positioned after a drop of anesthetic; read after 5 min.

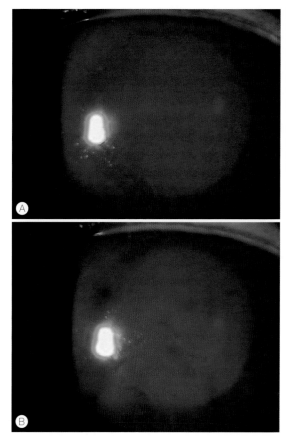

Fig. 2.2 Tear break-up time. (A) Immediately after administration of fluorescein: uniform distribution of dye, with no staining, and smooth surface. (B) Three seconds after: note "broken" areas of fluorescein, which appear as dark holes.

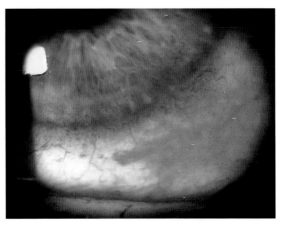

Fig. 2.3 Intense rose bengal staining in the inferior conjunctiva and peripheral cornea.

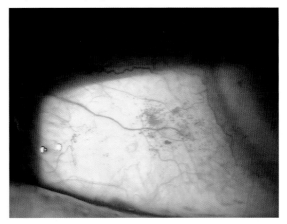

Fig. 2.4 Delicate rose bengal staining in the inferior conjunctiva and peripheral cornea.

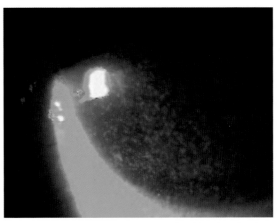

Fig. 2.5 Superficial punctate keratopathy; this alteration is often localized to the inferior cornea.

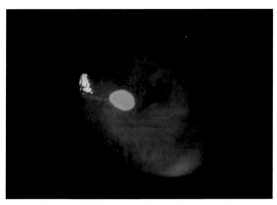

Fig. 2.6 Epithelial defect in a patient with severe dry eye: oval shape with clear margins and no infiltrate.

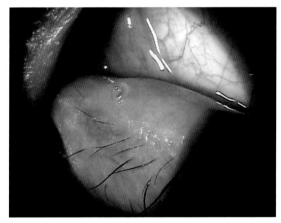

Fig. 2.7 Punctal plug (inferior punctum) in place.

Anterior Blepharitis

Key Facts

- Chronic ocular inflammation that primarily involves eyelashes and eyelid margin
- Common cause of chronic ocular irritation, including conjunctivitis, functional tear deficiency, and keratitis
- Staphylococcal and seborrheic are the most common causes
- Associated dry eye in 50–75% patients

Clinical Findings

- Irritation, redness, burning, watering, asthenopic symptoms
- Scaling and crusting along bases of eyelashes
- Loss of lashes, punctate epithelial erosions, neovascularization, and marginal infiltrates

Ancillary Testing

- Cultures of eyelid margins
- Assess dry eye status
- Biopsy of the eyelid (in areas of lash loss or persistent focal irritation)
- Microscopic evaluation of epilated eyelashes to look for *Demodex*

Differential Diagnosis

- Bacterial, viral, or parasitic infections
- Immunologic skin condition
- Allergic disorders
- Eyelid tumors
- Aqueous deficiency

Treatment

- Eyelid hygiene with warm compresses
- Topical antibiotics (e.g. erythromycin ointment)
- If significant inflammation, may require brief course of topical corticosteroid ointment to lid margins and eyelashes

Prognosis

- Chronic disease usually not sight-threatening but may lead to recurrent peripheral ulcers
- If untreated, eventual lash loss and lid scarring with trichiasis, corneal scarring, and neovascularization

SECTION 2 • Disorders of the Tear Film

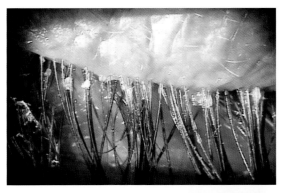

Fig. 2.8 Lid margin hyperemia, with crusting in lashes.

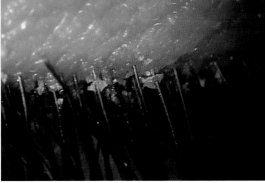

Fig. 2.9 Crusting along the cilia base: collarettes.

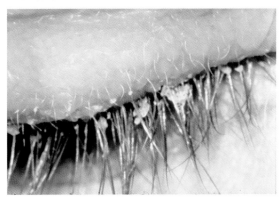

Fig. 2.10 Seborrheic blepharitis.

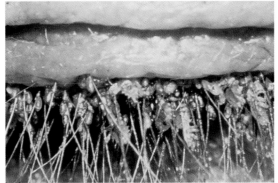

Fig. 2.11 Differential diagnosis: *Phthirus pubis* infestation.

Meibomian Gland Disease

Key Facts

- Also known as posterior blepharitis
- Frequently coexisting rosacea and seborrheic dermatitis
- Tear volume deficiency often associated
- Often associated with hordeola and chalazia

Clinical Findings

- Irritated or red eyes
- Thickened and erythematous lid margin
- Prominent blood vessels crossing mucocutaneous junction
- Pouting or plugging of meibomian orifices
- Poor expressibility and/or turbidity of meibomian secretions
- Dilation and eventual atrophy of meibomian glands
- Particulate, oily, or soapy debris in tear film

Ancillary Testing

- Fluorescein tear break-up time
- Corneal and conjunctival staining
- Biopsy of the eyelid if malignancy suspected

Differential Diagnosis

- Bacterial, viral, or parasitic infections
- Eyelid tumors

Treatment

- Eyelid hygiene
- Warm compresses followed by gentle massage
- Brief topical corticosteroid therapy
- Systemic tetracyclines
- Topical androgens or lipid supplements
- Dietary omega-3 fatty acid supplements

Prognosis

- Chronic disease, rarely sight-threatening
- Can be associated with hormonal balance and therefore may change as patient ages or becomes pregnant
- May lead to superficial punctate keratopathy, corneal neovascularization, and even stromal scarring

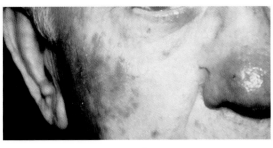

Fig. 2.12 Patient with rosacea.

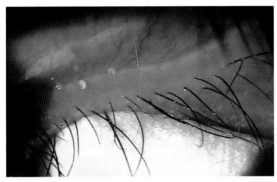

Fig. 2.13 Thickened meibomian gland secretion.

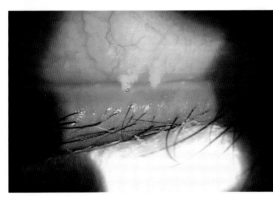

Fig. 2.14 Toothpaste-like meibomian gland secretion.

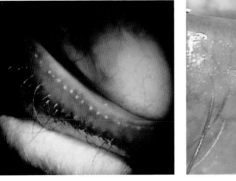

Fig. 2.15 Clogged meibomian gland orifices with turbidity of meibomian secretion.

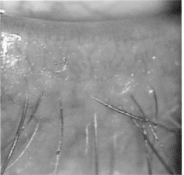

Fig. 2.16 Lid margin with prominent blood vessels and telangiectasia.

Filamentary Keratitis

Key Facts

- Desquamated epithelial cells and mucus adherent to corneal epithelium
- Chronic foreign body sensation
- Filaments' extremity moves with blink while the base does not; this pulling on the corneal stroma causes discomfort
- More common in superior aspect of the cornea
- **Etiologies include:**
  - dry eyes • occlusion • viral infection • lid abnormalities • superior limbic keratoconjunctivitis

Clinical Findings

- Corneal filaments are adherent to the underlying stroma at one focal point and appear as a vertical strand that moves with blinking
- Stain with fluorescein dye

Ancillary Testing

- Evaluation of dry eye including Schirmer testing
- Fluorescein and rose bengal staining
- Evaluation of superior limbus for gelatinous thickening of limbal tissue and horizontal vascular engorgement to look for superior limbic keatoconjunctivitis
- Assessment of lid position, chronic occlusion, or numerous medications

Differential Diagnosis

- Superior limbic keratoconjunctivitis
- Keratoconjunctivitis sicca
- Long-term occlusion
- Recurrent erosion
- Bullous keratopathy
- Herpes simplex
- Medicamentosa
- Ptosis

Treatment

- Removal of filaments at base with forceps at the slit lamp under topical anesthesia
- Treatment of underlying keratoconjunctivitis sicca with supplemental lubrication or punctal occlusion
- Surgical management of ptosis
- Surgical management of occlusion
- Avoidance of ointments
- Topical low-dose corticosteroid such as fluorometholone
- Consider conjunctival resection if secondary to superior limbic keratoconjunctivitis
- Consider collagenase inhibitor (Acetylcysteine [Mucomyst] 10% q.i.d.)

Prognosis

- Good if underlying etiology identified and treated
- May progress in severe keratoconjunctivitis sicca
- May recur in superior limbic keratoconjunctivitis

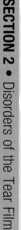

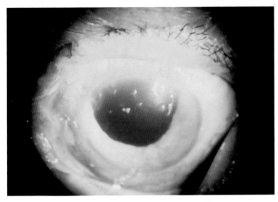

Fig. 2.17 Corneal filaments in a patient with Sjögren syndrome; they should be promptly removed.

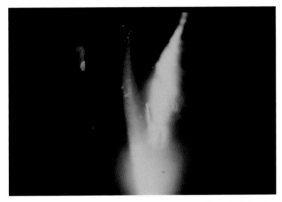

Fig. 2.18 Inferior filaments. They can be small and delicate, and the examiner should perform a detailed slit-lamp examination.

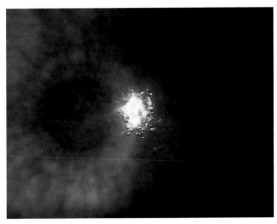

Fig. 2.19 Corneal epithelial rough surface with loss of luster and central filaments.

Section 3
Conjunctiva

Adult Bacterial (Non-gonococcal) Conjunctivitis

Key Facts

- Diagnosis classically based on history and clinical picture
- Frequently bilateral and asymmetric
- Most cases caused by gram-positive bacteria
- **Risk factors include:**
  - contact with infected persons • infection or abnormality of adnexal structure
    - severe tear deficiency • immunosuppression • trauma

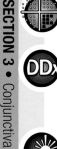

Clinical Findings

- Bulbar conjunctival injection
- Purulent or mucopurulent discharge
- Conjunctival membranes and/or pseudomembranes
- Papillary hypertrophy or rare follicular hyperplasia

Ancillary Testing

- Gram stain
- Cultures

Differential Diagnosis

- Allergic conjunctivitis
- Viral conjunctivitis
- Canaliculitis
- Blepharitis

Treatment

- Broad-spectrum topical antibiotic (e.g. an aminoglycoside, trimethoprim–polymixin B [Polytrim], or a fluoroquinolone) is the first-line treatment
  - may be altered if lack of clinical response based on culture results
- Maintain proper ocular and periocular hygiene

Prognosis

- Usually self-limited in adults
- Rare complications include keratitis, corneal opacities, and periorbital cellulitis
- Economic impact of the disease, in terms of lost work time, is considerable

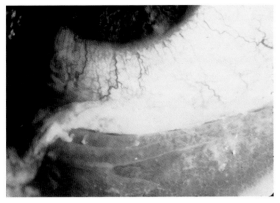

Fig. 3.1 Purulent discharge, chemosis, and diffuse hyperemia. *Streptococcus pneumoniae* was the cultured organism.

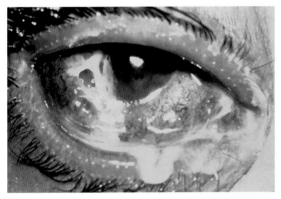

Fig. 3.2 Copious mucopurulent discharge and pronounced chemosis in a patient with acute bacterial conjunctivitis.

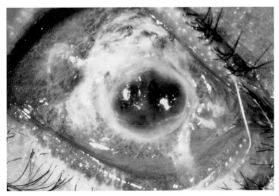

Fig. 3.3 Gonococcal conjunctivitis: corneal melting.

Adenoviral Keratoconjunctivitis

Key Facts

- Self-limited infection (resolution usually within 5–7 days but can persist for ≤2 weeks)
- Unilateral or bilateral
- Exposed surfaces can be decontaminated by wiping with 2% sodium hypochlorite or household chlorine bleach 1 : 10 dilution with water

Clinical Findings

- Conjunctival injection
- Watery discharge
- Follicular reaction of conjunctiva is clinical hallmark
- **Distinctive or often found signs:**
  - preauricular lymphadenopathy • subconjunctival hemorrhage • corneal epithelial erosion • multifocal epithelial punctate keratitis evolving to anterior stromal keratitis
- Chronic subepithelial infiltrates in some patients

Ancillary Testing

- Cultures
- PCR
- Both are rarely needed—clinical diagnosis is often easily done

Differential Diagnosis

- Toxic, allergic, bacterial, or chlamydial conjunctivitis
- Canaliculitis
- Blepharitis

Treatment

- Wash hands frequently, use separate towels, and avoid close contact with others during period of contagion (10–14 days after onset)
- Cold compresses
- Topical steroids in severe cases of keratoconjunctivitis (subepithelial infiltrates)—controversial
- Debridement of membranes
- Use of antiviral agents is under clinical investigation

Prognosis

- Usually non–sight-threatening condition
- Economic impact of the disease, in terms of lost work time, is considerable
- Subepithelial infiltrates can cause temporary decreased vision
- Postviral keratoconjunctivitis sicca is possible

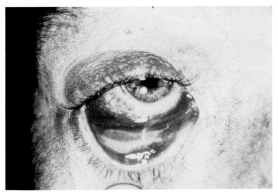

Fig. 3.4 Conjunctival hyperemia with pseudomembrane on the inferior tarsal conjunctiva.

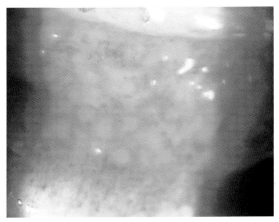

Fig. 3.5 Multiple conjunctival follicles.

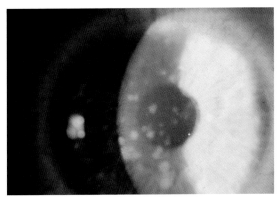

Fig. 3.6 Corneal subepithelial infiltrates in epidemic viral keratoconjunctivitis.

Adenoviral Keratoconjunctivitis (Continued)

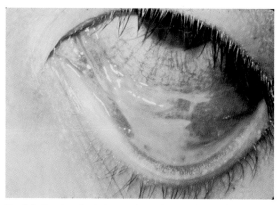

Fig. 3.7 Conjunctival chemosis and pseudomembrane.

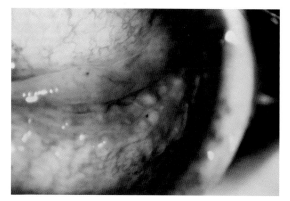

Fig. 3.8 Conjunctival follicles.

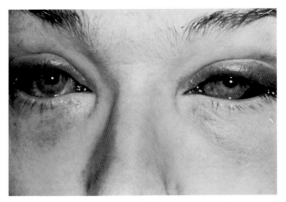

Fig. 3.9 Bilateral involvement: diffuse conjunctival hyperemia and chemosis. Note also the swollen eyelids.

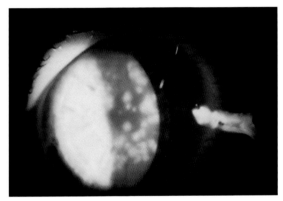

Fig. 3.10 Corneal subepithelial infiltrates in epidemic viral keratoconjunctivitis.

Adult Inclusion (Chlamydial) Conjunctivitis

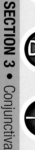

Key Facts

- *Chlamydia trachomatis* serotypes D–K
- Most common in sexually active young adults
- Oculogenital spread or other intimate contact with infected person

Clinical Findings

- Bulbar conjunctival injection
- Follicular reaction (prominent and well developed) of tarsal conjunctiva (especially inferior fornices)
- Mild mucoid discharge
- Ipsilateral preauricular lymphadenopathy
- Subepithelial infiltrates in later stages

Ancillary Testing

- Conjunctical scrapings for Giemsa and culture (McCoy cell media)
- PCR
- Direct immunofluorescent antibody test

Differential Diagnosis

- Viral, adenoviral, or bacterial infection
- Allergic or toxic reaction
- Early stage trachoma

Treatment

- **Systemic therapy is indicated:**
  - azithromycin 1 g orally single dose *or*
  - doxycycline 100 mg orally twice a day for 3 weeks
- Treat sexual partners

Prognosis

- Frequently no sequelae
- Rarely conjunctival scarring, corneal pannus, scarring, and neovascularization

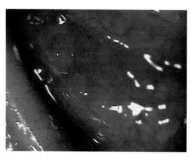

Fig. 3.11 Large follicles on the inferior tarsal conjunctiva: a typical finding.

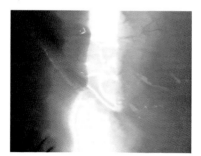

Fig. 3.12 Large follicles on inferior tarsal conjunctiva: a typical finding.

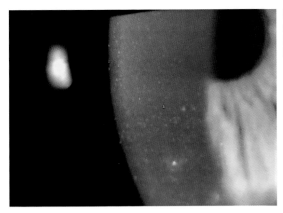

Fig. 3.13 Corneal superficial (subepithelial) infiltrate.

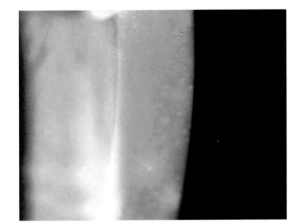

Fig. 3.14 Corneal superficial (subepithelial) infiltrate in detail.

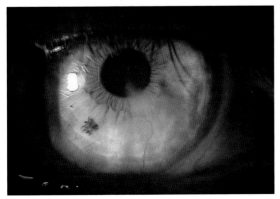

Fig. 3.15 Corneal superficial neovascularization due to chlamydial chronic conjunctivitis.

Trachoma

Key Facts

- Most common infectious cause of blindness worldwide (5.9 million people)
- More common in poor communities, with a heterogeneous distribution
- Trachomatous inflammation follicular and trachomatous inflammation intense are most common in young children
- Trachomatous trichiasis represents serious risk of corneal opacity and vision loss and is more prevalent in women
- **Endemic areas:**
    - Africa • Middle East • Central and South America • Asia • Australia • Pacific Islands
- Etiologic factor is an obligate intracellular bacteria, *Chlamydia trachomatis* (serotypes A, B, Ba, and C)
- Incubation period of 5–10 days, manifests as chronic keratoconjunctivitis (repeated infections)

Clinical Findings

- Subepithelial follicles (hallmark of active disease) and papillary hypertrophy in tarsal conjunctiva
- Superficial punctate keratitis or vascular infiltration of superior cornea (pannus)
- Herbert pits (depressions at upper limbus caused by replacement of follicles by scar)
- Arlt line (fibrosis leading to scarring in upper tarsal conjunctiva)
- Trichiasis or entropion
- Corneal opacity and neovascularization

Ancillary Testing

- In general, the diagnosis is made on clinical and epidemiologic data
- Tissue culture, immunofluorescence, ELISA, PCR

Differential Diagnosis

- Other bacterial and/or viral conjunctivitis • Vernal keratoconjunctivitis
    - Mucous membrane pemphigoid or Stevens–Johnson syndrome

Treatment

- SAFE strategy (proposed by the World Health Organization)
    - Surgery for lid abnormalities: tarsal rotation, epilation • Antibiotic for active disease: single-dose oral azithromycin 1 g or tetracycline ointment b.i.d. for 6 weeks • Facial cleanliness: dirty faces are associated with trachoma • Environmental improvement: activities to control trachoma are interventions undertaken with the community rather than treatment for persons in medical facilities

Prognosis

- Poor if lid disease is not treated, resulting in corneal scarring, neovascularization, and vision loss
- Conjunctival scarring leads to loss of goblet cells and limbal stem cells, leading to secondary dry eye and stem cell deficiency with pannus
- Secondary infection (bacteria or fungi) of traumatized cornea may occur

World Health Organization Simplified Grading System For Trachoma

- TF (trachomatous inflammation, follicular): presence of five or more follicles of ≥0.5 mm diameter in central part of upper tarsal conjunctiva
- TI (trachomatous inflammation, intense): pronounced inflammatory thickening of upper tarsal conjunctiva obscuring more than half of the normal deep tarsal vessels
- TS (trachomatous conjunctival scarring): presence of easily visible scars in tarsal conjunctiva
- TT (trachomatous trichiasis): at least one eyelash rubbing on the eyeball or evidence of recent removal of in-turned eyelashes
- CO (corneal opacity): easily visible corneal opacity over the pupil, so dense that at least part of the pupil margin is blurred when viewed through the opacity

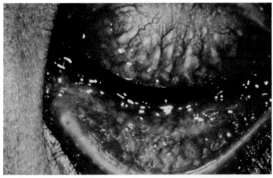

Fig. 3.16 Conjunctival diffuse tarsal involvement: follicular conjunctivitis.

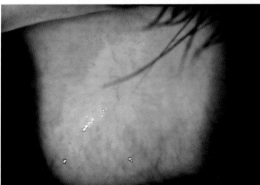

Fig. 3.17 Subepithelial line of scarring in superior tarsal conjunctiva.

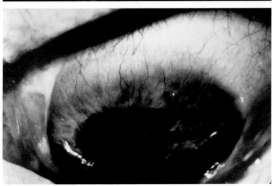

Fig. 3.18 Herbert pits and peripheral pannus: a pathognomonic sign.

Molluscum Conjunctivitis

Key Facts
- Dermatotropic DNA poxvirus
- Humans are the only host
- More common in children and young adults (especially HIV-infected patients)
- Spread by close personal contact, can be sexually transmitted

Clinical Findings
- Chronic follicular conjunctivitis
- Pink, umbilicated lesions on lid margin
- Superficial punctate keratitis

Ancillary Testing
- Often a clinical diagnosis
- Histopathologic examination can show eosinophilic intracytoplasmic inclusion bodies (Henderson–Patterson bodies)

Differential Diagnosis
- Herpes simplex
- Verruca vulgaris (human papillomavirus)
- Keratoachantoma (early stages)
- Adenovirus—after all, molluscum typically presents as a monocular follicular conjunctivitis

Treatment
- Surgical removal (excision or curettage)
- Cryotherapy of lesions

Prognosis
- May resolve spontaneously (months to years) in immunocompetent patients
- Occasionally lesions may become secondarily infected
- Rarely secondary corneal pannus

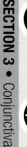

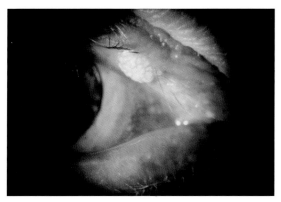

Fig. 3.19 Molluscum eyelid lesion.

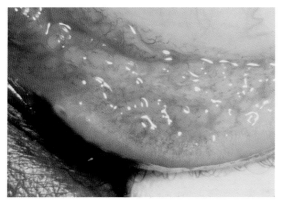

Fig. 3.20 Follicular conjunctivitis secondary to molluscum infection.

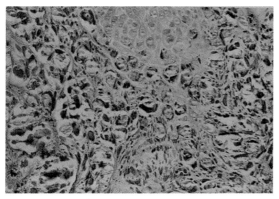

Fig. 3.21 Histopathologic examination: eosinophilic intracytoplasmic inclusion (Henderson–Patterson) bodies.

Allergic (Seasonal and Perennial) Conjunctivitis

Key Facts

- Type 1 allergic response
- Classically associated with allergic rhinitis
- Most prevalent form of ocular allergy
- Hallmark symptom is itching

Clinical Findings

- Photophobia, tearing, burning
- Conjunctival hyperemia
- Mildpapillary reaction
- Chemosis
- Clear and stringy discharge

Ancillary Testing

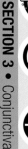

- Allergen skin testing (prick or intradermal methods)
- Conjunctival scrapings or impression cytology

Differential Diagnosis

- Blepharitis
- Toxic reaction
- Adenoviral conjunctivitis

Treatment

- Avoid known allergens
- Topical antihistamines, steroids (judicious use), and mast cell stabilizers
- Artificial tears
- Cold compresses
- Avoid eye rubbing, which can result in histamine release from mast cells

Prognosis

- Can cause significant morbidity
- Rarely sight-threatening

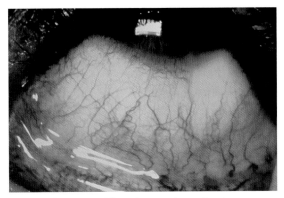

Fig. 3.22 Chemosis, diffuse hyperemia, and watery discharge. The main complaint was itching.

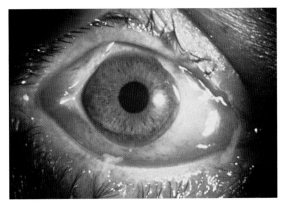

Fig. 3.23 Seasonal allergic conjunctivitis with severe chemosis. (Courtesy of W. Barry Lee, MD.)

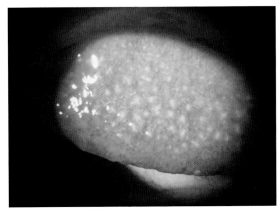

Fig. 3.24 Papillary reaction on superior tarsal conjunctiva. (Courtesy of W. Barry Lee, MD.)

Giant Papillary Conjunctivitis

Key Facts

- **Non-infectious, chronic inflammatory process related to:**
  - mechanical trauma
  - repeat immunologic presentation
- **Occurs in relation to:**
  - contact lens wear (most common) • exposed sutures • glaucoma filtering blebs • ocular prosthetics • band keratopathy • extruded scleral buckles

Clinical Findings

- Mild hyperemia
- Scant mucous discharge
- Papillary hypertrophy (>1.5 mm diameter), mostly on superior tarsal conjunctiva
- Fluorescein staining of apex of papillae

Ancillary Testing

- Diagnosis made with clinical history and slit-lamp examination

Differential Diagnosis

- Allergic, vernal, or atopic conjunctivitis
- Blepharitis
- Toxic conjunctivitis
- Foreign body

Treatment

- Removal of inciting agent until symptoms have resolved
  - Inactive giant papillae may persist long after active inflammation has resolved
- Change patient's contact lens care
- Topical steroids restricted to acute phases

Prognosis

- Permanent visual loss never reported

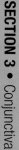

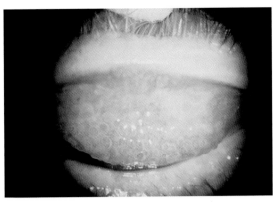

Fig. 3.25 Giant papillae (>1.5 mm) in the superior tarsal conjunctiva of a long-term contact lens wearer.

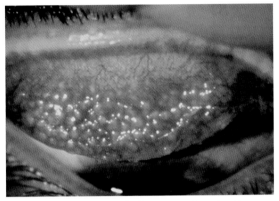

Fig. 3.26 Another case of GPC due to soft contact lens wear.

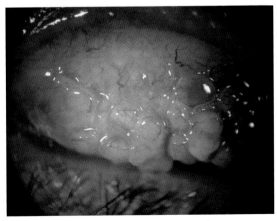

Fig. 3.27 Giant papillary conjunctivitis secondary to an exposed nylon suture (superior trabeculectomy). (Courtesy of the External Eye Disease and Cornea Section, Federal University of Sao Paulo, Brazil.)

Vernal Conjunctivitis

Key Facts

- More common in younger ages and in males
- More prevalent in hot and dry environments
- Associated with keratoconus (probably secondary to chronic eye rubbing)
- **Main symptoms:**
  - itching • photophobia • foreign body sensation • tearing

Clinical Findings

- Thick mucous discharge
- Bulbar conjunctival injection
- Marked papillary response, mainly on limbus and superior tarsal conjunctiva
- Horner–Trantas dots (macroaggregates of degenerated eosinophils and epithelial cells)
- Punctate epithelial keratitis, epithelial erosions, shield ulcer

Ancillary Testing

- Tear fluid analysis and cytology
- Conjunctival scrapings for cytology

Differential Diagnosis

- Atopic conjunctivitis

Treatment

- Avoidance of allergens
- Topical steroids (short-term, high-dose pulse regimen)
- Topical mast cell stabilizer
- Topical cyclosporin A
- Antibiotics with steroids in shield ulcers

Prognosis

- Can be sight-threatening
- Usually remission occurs after puberty

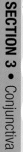

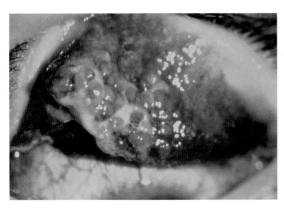

Fig. 3.28 Giant papillae in the superior tarsal conjunctiva, mucous discharge, and corneal shield ulcer in a young boy with vernal keratoconjunctivitis.

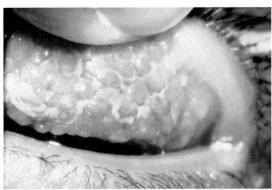

Fig. 3.29 Giant papillae and copious mucous discharge in the superior tarsal conjunctiva.

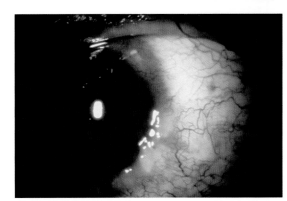

Fig. 3.30 Cobblestone papillae. Note size and flattened surface due to permanent contact with the globe.

Fig. 3.31 Gelatinous appearance of limbal follicles and Trantas dots.

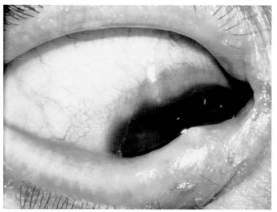

Fig. 3.32 Limbal form of vernal keratoconjunctivitis.

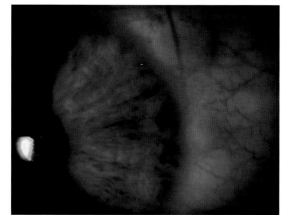

Fig. 3.33 Trantas dots stained with fluorescein.

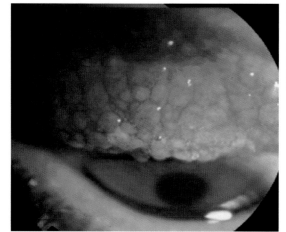

Fig. 3.34 Palpebral form, with giant cobblestone papillae (same patient as in Fig. 3.33).

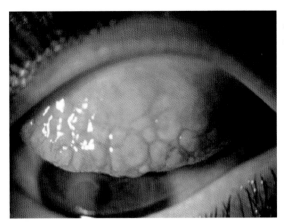

Fig. 3.35 Palpebral form, with giant cobblestone papillae (same patient as in Fig. 3.33).

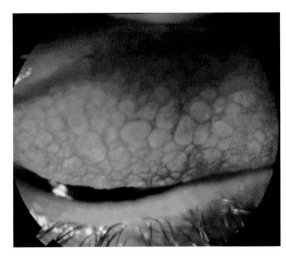

Fig. 3.36 Palpebral form, with giant cobblestone papillae (same patient as in Fig. 3.33).

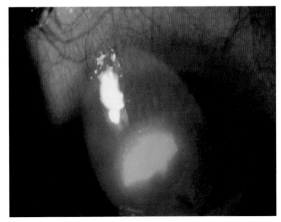

Fig. 3.37 Shield ulcer stained with fluorescein. Note oval shape and clean borders. No evidence of bacterial superinfection.

Atopic Conjunctivitis

Key Facts

- Bilateral disease
- Associated with atopic dermatitis
- Onset usually in second through fifth decades
- No racial or geographic predilection but genetic predisposition to atopy
- Higher risk of herpetic keratitis

Clinical Findings

- **Symptoms include:**
  - itching • watering • blurred vision • photophobia
- Periocular dermatitis and lid thickening
- Conjunctival hyperemia, pale white chemosis, subepithelial fibrosis
- Papillary and follicular reaction on tarsal surfaces
- Lids alterations, which can develop to cicatricial ectropion and lagophthalmos
- Eczematoid blepharitis, loss of cilia, meibomitis, punctal ectropion

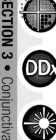

Ancillary Testing

- Conjunctival scrapings or impression cytology
- Biopsy

Differential Diagnosis

- Vernal conjunctivitis
- Ocular cicatricial pemphigoid

Treatment

- Environmental control of allergens
- Topical steroids (judicious use), antihistamines, and mast cell stabilizers
- Cyclosporin A (both topical and systemic)
- Surgical correction of lid and ocular surface abnormalities

Prognosis

- Challenging, sight-threatening condition

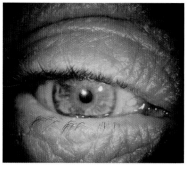

Fig. 3.38 Thickened and swollen eyelids.

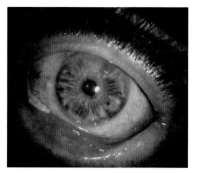

Fig. 3.39 Same patient as in Fig. 3.38, with mucous discharge and diffuse conjunctival hyperemia.

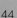

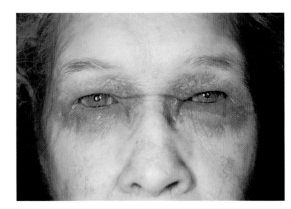

Fig. 3.40 Atopic conjunctivitis: patient's facial skin showing periocular dermatitis.

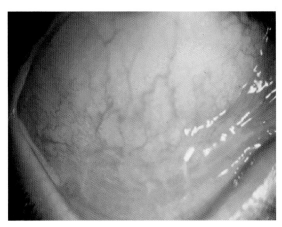

Fig. 3.41 Chemosis, conjunctival hyperemia, and subconjunctival scarring. Chronic disease can lead to fornix shortening.

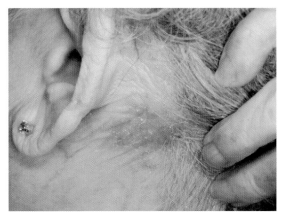

Fig. 3.42 Skin lesion in a patient with atopic disease.

Ocular Cicatricial Pemphigoid (Mucous Membrane Pemphigoid)

Key Facts

- Chronic systemic autoimmune disease
- Deposition of immunoglobulins and complement in conjunctival basement membrane zone
- More common in elderly people (average age at onset is 65 years) and women
- No racial or geographic predilection
- Association with other autoimmune diseases (e.g. rheumatoid arthritis)

Clinical Findings

- Keratoconjunctivitis sicca
- Subepithelial fibrosis and fornix foreshortening
- Symblepharon or ankyloblepharon
- Entropion, trichiasis, dystichiasis, lagophthalmos
- Corneal pannus, pseudopterygium, corneal scarring, keratinization of ocular surface

Ancillary Testing

- Conjunctival biopsy and immunohistochemistry

Differential Diagnosis

- Atopic conjunctivitis
- Ocular rosacea
- Chemical burn
- Stevens–Johnson syndrome
- Linear IgA disease
- Pseudo (drug-induced) ocular cicatricial pemphigoid

Treatment

- Systemic immunomodulation
  - dapsone • corticosteroids • azathioprine • methotrexate • mycophenolate mofetil • cyclophosphamide
- **Ocular:**
  - punctal plugs • intense lubrication • lid and corneal surgeries, including keratoprosthesis in advanced cases (*requires adequate immunomodulation*)

Prognosis

- Chronic and slow progression that often leads to eventual bilateral blindness
- Therapy can only arrest scarring but not reverse it and is associated with a number of systemic and ocular complications
- Risk of potentially lethal complications (tracheal and esophageal strictures)

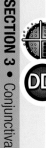

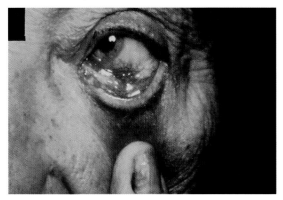

Fig. 3.43 Symblepharon formation in stage 1 disease. Note conjunctival inflammation.

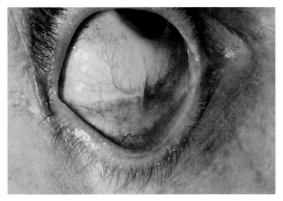

Fig. 3.44 Inferior fornix shortening and symblepharon. The disease is under control and without conjunctival inflammation at this time.

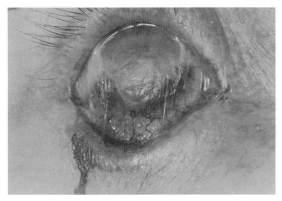

Fig. 3.45 Advanced disease, with keratinization of the cornea and ocular surface.

Modified Foster Grading System

- Stage 1: subepithelial fibrosis without foreshortening of fornix
- Stage 2: fornix foreshortening
  A (0–25%)
  B (25–50%)
  C (50–75%)
  D (>75%)
- Stage 3: presence of symblepharon
  A (0–25%)
  B (25–50%)
  C (50–75%)
  D (>75%)
- Stage 4: ankyloblepharon and ocular surface keratinization

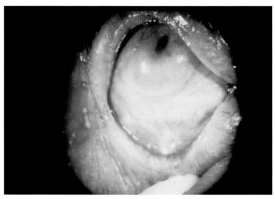

Fig. 3.46 Inferior fornix shortening and symblepharon, thickened eyelid margins.

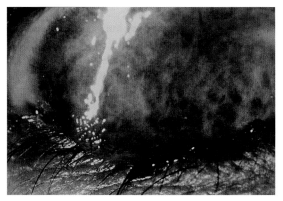

Fig. 3.47 Subepithelial fibrosis and scarring of the superior tarsal conjunctiva.

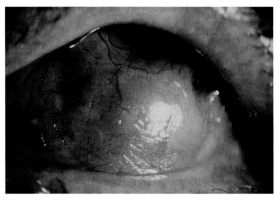

Fig. 3.48 End stage disease: corneal scarring, neovascularization, and keratinization; guarded visual prognosis.

Ocular Cicatricial Pemphigoid (continued)

Stevens–Johnson Syndrome

Key Facts

- Systemic reaction to certain drugs or infections
  Drugs most commonly associated:
  - antimicrobials (sulfonamides, penicillins, cephalosporins, others)
    - anticonvulsants • metals • non-steroidal anti-inflammatory drugs
      - cardiovascular drugs
  Infections most commonly associated:
  - herpes simplex • *Mycoplasma pneumoniae* • measles • *Mycobacterium*
    - group A streptococci • Epstein–Barr virus • *Yersinia* • enterovirus
      - smallpox vaccination
- Estimated incidence is 1.1–7.1 cases/million persons per year
- Ocular and dermatologic signs can begin 1–3 weeks after initial exposure
- Target skin lesions (<3 cm)
- At least two areas of mucous membrane involvement

Clinical Findings

- **Acute phase:**
  - bilateral non-specific conjunctivitis • anterior uveitis
- **Chronic phase:**
  - dry eye, scarring, symblepharon • entropion, trichiasis • destruction of limbal stem cells, leading to corneal scarring, neovascularization, and perforation

Ancillary Testing

- Complete blood count, systemic evaluation
- Conjunctival biopsy or impression cytology

Differential Diagnosis

- Atopic conjunctivitis
- Ocular cicatricial pemphigoid
- Trachoma
- Chemical burns

Treatment

- **Systemic:** supportive care (sometimes in critical care or burn units)
- Ocular
  Acute phase:
  - ocular hygiene, prophylatic antibiotics, cycloplegics
  Chronic phase:
  - lid or fornix reconstruction
  - treat dry eye aggressively
  - keratolimbal allograft and penetrating keratoplasty have a low rate of success secondary to severe dry eye and conjunctival scarring

Prognosis

- Potentially fatal disease
- Ocular disease severity depends on severity of initial event
- Some patients can develop recurrent conjunctival inflammation
- Prevalence of lifelong disability from ocular morbidity has remained unchanged for past 35 years

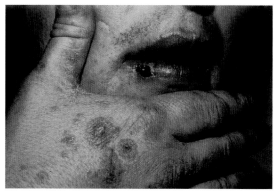

Fig. 3.49 Typical skin lesions.

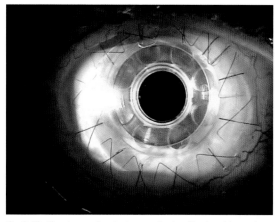

Fig. 3.50 Keratoprosthesis in a patient with visual loss due to Stevens–Johnson syndrome. The vision was 20/30.

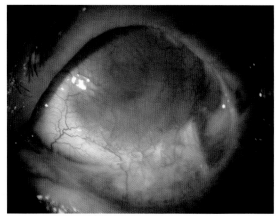

Fig. 3.51 Corneal neovascularization and scarring with associated symblepharon and cicatrizing conjunctival changes. (Courtesy of the External Eye Disease and Cornea Section, Federal University of Sao Paulo, Brazil.)

Superior Limbic Keratoconjunctivitis

Key Facts

- Inflammation of superior tarsal and bulbar conjunctiva
- Probably arises from blink-related microtrauma
- Association with thyroid autoimmune diseases
- Unilateral or bilateral

Clinical Findings

- Dilation of superior bulbar conjunctival blood vessels
- Superior bulbar conjunctival hyperemia and chemosis
- Redundant superior bulbar conjunctiva
- Papillary reaction on superior tarsal conjunctiva
- Corneal superior micropannus and filaments
- Thick eyelid margin or ptosis

Ancillary Testing

- Superior bulbar conjunctival and limbal staining with fluorescein and rose bengal
- Biopsy

Differential Diagnosis

- Reaction to cosmetic soft contact lenses (contact lens–induced keratoconjunctivitis)
- Dry eye
- Allergic or toxic conjunctivitis

Treatment

- Control thyroid disease if present
- Lubricating agents or punctal plugs
- Topical vitamin A, cyclosporin A, silver nitrate solution
- Mast cell–stabilizing agents, topical steroids (judicious use), autologous serum
- Therapeutic contact lens, pressure patching
- Sectorial resection or thermal cauterization of affected bulbar conjunctiva

Prognosis

- Good visual prognosis
- Multiple recurrences and remissions can occur

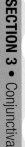

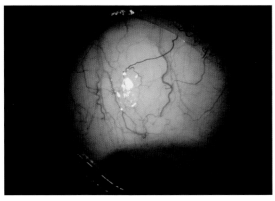

Fig. 3.52 Engorged vessels and mild inflammation; these changes were localized on the superior bulbar conjunctiva.

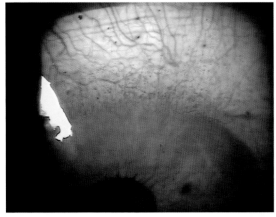

Fig. 3.53 Typical aspect of rose bengal staining. Redundant bulbar conjunctiva.

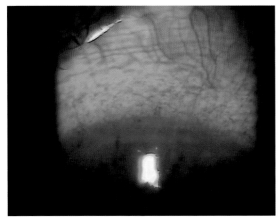

Fig. 3.54 Typical aspect of fluorescein staining. Corneal superior micropannus. Check for fluorescein staining on the superior bulbar conjunctiva.

Phlyctenular Keratoconjunctivitis

Key Facts

- Allergic cell-mediated response (type 4)
- **Main etiologies:**
  - tuberculosis • staphylococcal blepharitis • worm infestation
- More common in younger patients

Clinical Findings

- Phlyctenule (more common at limbus)
- Conjunctival injection, discharge, nodules, ulceration
- Corneal ulceration or neovascularization
- Corneal scars

Ancillary Testing

- **Investigate the specific etiology:**
  - lid margin and conjunctival swabs (staphylococcal blepharitis)
  - stool examination (worms)
  - chest x-ray, purified protein derivative, complete blood count (tuberculosis)

Differential Diagnosis

- Allergic vernal conjunctivitis
- Salzmann degeneration nodules
- Infectious keratitis
- Nodular episcleritis

Treatment

- Topical steroid–antibiotic combination
- Treat specific etiology

Prognosis

- Recurrences more common in tuberculosis
- Visual impairment not uncommon
- Rarely leads to blindness

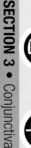

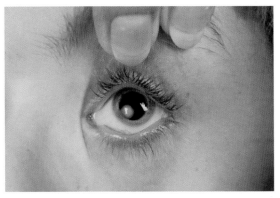

Fig. 3.55 Boy with phlyctenular keratoconjunctivitis due to chronic staphylococcal blepharitis.

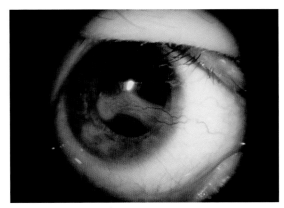

Fig. 3.56 Typical aspect: superficial neovascularization and opacity.

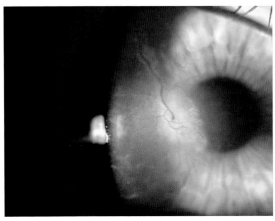

Fig. 3.57 Another example with similar findings.

Conjunctival Intraepithelial Neoplasia

Key Facts

- Involves epithelium only (without penetrating basement membrane)
- More common in white males
- Human papillomavirus infection is a well-known risk factor
- Frequently asymptomatic
- Usually found at limbus in interpalpebral fissure

Clinical Findings

- Fleshy gelatinous lesion, usually at limbus
- Can be sessile or minimally elevated
- A white plaque (leukoplakia) can occur at the lesion's surface
- Fine vessels

Ancillary Testing

- Excisional biopsy (can be the definitive treatment)
- Exfoliative cytology

Differential Diagnosis

- Invasive squamous cell carcinoma
- Nevus
- Pingueculae
- Bitot spot (vitamin A deficiency)

Treatment

- Excisional biopsy
- Surgical removal (partial lamellar sclerokeratoconjunctivectomy) and cryotherapy
- Topical chemotherapy (mitomycin-C or 5-fluorouracil)
- Recommended that an incisional biopsy be done before chemotherapy treatment

Prognosis

- No metastatic potential
- Can rarely progress to invasive squamous cell carcinoma
- Recurrences are common, especially with excisional biopsy without adjunctive treatment

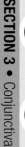

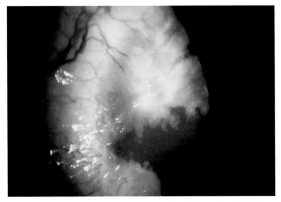

Fig. 3.58 Limbal conjunctival intraepithelial neoplasia: fleshy gelatinous, elevated lesion.

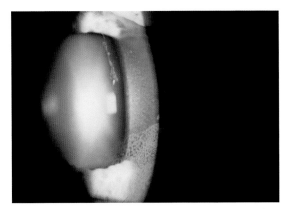

Fig. 3.59 Same patient as in Fig. 3.58, showing corneal spread. Definitive diagnosis after excisional biopsy.

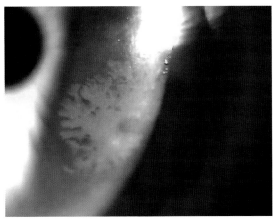

Fig. 3.60 Corneal involvement: typical aspect.

Squamous Cell Carcinoma

Key Facts

- Extension of tumor through basement membrane
- **Related to:**
  - human papillomavirus infection • sun exposure • smoking
- Immunosuppressed patients at higher risk of aggressive and bilateral disease
- Usually found at limbus in interpalpebral fissure
- Pigmentation may be present

Clinical Findings

- Fleshy gelatinous lesion, usually at limbus
- Can be sessile or minimally elevated
- A white plaque (leukoplakia) can occur at the lesion's surface
- Engorged feeder vessels

Ancillary Testing

- Excisional biopsy (can be the definitive treatment)
- Exfoliative cytology
- Ultrasonography

Differential Diagnosis

- Conjunctival intraepithelial neoplasia
- Pinguecula
- Pterygium
- Mucoepidermoid carcinoma

Treatment

- Excisional biopsy
- Surgical removal (partial lamellar sclerokeratoconjunctivectomy) and cryotherapy
- Topical chemotherapy (mitomycin-C or 5-fluorouracil)

Prognosis

- Can invade the eye and soft tissues adjacent to the globe
- Can metastasize to regional (preauricular and submandibular) lymph nodes (uncommon)

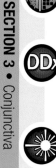

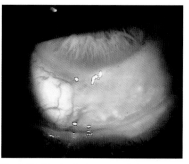

Fig. 3.61 Fleshy lesion on inferior bulbar conjunctiva.

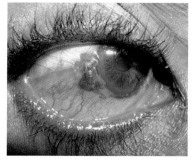

Fig. 3.62 Squamous cell carcinoma. This elevated lesion in the temporal limbus shows a keratinized surface and secondary acquired melanosis. (Courtesy of Bruno F. Fernandes, MD.)

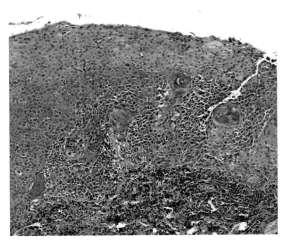

Fig. 3.63 Squamous cell carcinoma. Atypical epithelial cells occupying the entire epithelium and invading the basement membrane. Stromal inflammation and collections of keratinized cells (horn pearls) are also seen. Periodic acid Schiff, ×100. (Courtesy of Bruno F. Fernandes, MD, and Miguel N. Burnier Jr., MD, PhD.)

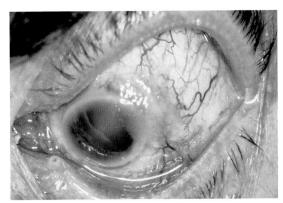

Fig. 3.64 Large limbal lesion with diffuse vascularization and inflammation.

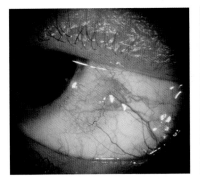

Fig. 3.65 Limbal lesion with engorged feeder vessels.

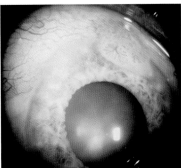

Fig. 3.66 Superior limbal involvement with corneal spread.

Primary Acquired Melanosis

Key Facts

- Can occur anywhere but usually located at bulbar conjunctiva
- Benign condition (affects epithelium), malignant potential
- Often unilateral, acquired in middle age
- Pigmentation can wax and wane over time
- One-third of white patients have primary acquired melanosis to some degree

Clinical Findings

- Brown lesion with ill-defined margins
- Flat, patchy lesion
- Non-cystic

Ancillary Testing

- Diagnostic biopsy
- Photographic documentation, although non-malignant lesions will still change shape and location over time

Differential Diagnosis

- Nevus
- Racial melanosis
- Melanoma

Treatment

- Periodic observation
- Complete excisional biopsy and cryotherapy
- Topical chemotherapy with mitomycin-C

Prognosis

- If no cellular atypia, the risk to malignant progression does not exist
- Progress to melanoma in ≤50% of cases with cellular atypia

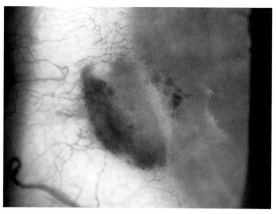

Fig. 3.67 Primary acquired melanosis. Flat pigmented lesion that advanced into the cornea. (Courtesy of Bruno F. Fernandes, MD.)

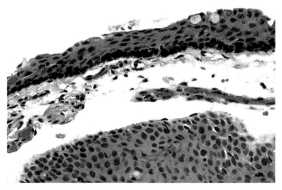

Fig. 3.68 Primary acquired melanosis without atypia: basilar hyperplasia of typical melanocytes. Hematoxylin and eosin, ×400. (Courtesy of Bruno F. Fernandes, MD, and Miguel N. Burnier Jr., MD, PhD.)

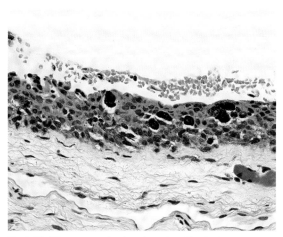

Fig. 3.69 Primary acquired melanosis with atypia: presence of atypical melanocytes within the superficial layers of the epithelium. Hematoxylin and eosin, ×400. (Courtesy of Bruno F. Fernandes, MD, and Miguel N. Burnier Jr., MD, PhD.)

Conjunctival Nevus

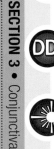

Key Facts

- Classically located at interpalpebral limbus
- Almost always unilateral
- Can become thicker and more pigmented over time, especially during puberty
- Becomes clinically apparent in first or second decade
- Most common melanocytic conjunctival tumor

Clinical Findings

- Slightly elevated, sessile lesion
- Can have brown or yellow color
- Cysts found in many patients
- Well-defined margins

Ancillary Testing

- Diagnostic biopsy
- Photographic documentation
- Exfoliative cytology

Differential Diagnosis

- Melanoma
- Primary acquired melanosis
- Racial melanosis

Treatment

- Periodic observation
- Surgical excision for cosmetic reasons

Prognosis

- Benign lesion—vision loss does not occur
- <1% progress to melanoma (higher risk in white people than in African Americans)

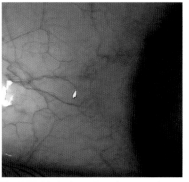

Fig. 3.70 Limbal amelanotic nevus in a 16-year-old girl.

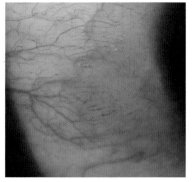

Fig. 3.71 Higher magnification of the nevus in Fig. 3.70, showing intralesional cysts.

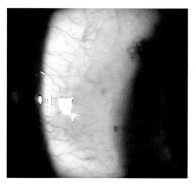

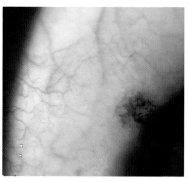

Fig. 3.72 Slightly elevated, pigmented nevus on superior limbus.

Fig. 3.73 Detailed image of the nevus in Fig. 3.72: well-defined margins and intralesional cysts.

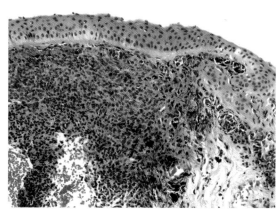

Fig. 3.74 Compound conjunctival nevus: junctional nests of nevus cells and a deep subepithelial component. Note maturation of cells at the base of the lesion. Hematoxylin and eosin, ×200. (Courtesy of Bruno F. Fernandes, MD, and Miguel N. Burnier Jr., MD, PhD.)

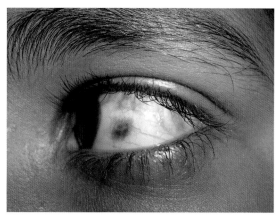

Fig. 3.75 Conjunctival nevus. Flat pigmented lesion on the bulbar conjunctiva, containing epithelial inclusion cysts. (Courtesy of Bruno F. Fernandes, MD.)

Conjunctival Melanoma

Key Facts

- Can occur anywhere in bulbar or palpebral conjunctiva
- Usually unilateral brown or pink lesion (may be non-pigmented [amelanotic])
- Most commonly arises from primary acquired melanosis (PAM)
- Typically affects white adults

Clinical Findings

- Usually well-defined margins
- Can be pigmented, amelanotyc, or tan-colored
- Vascularized nodule
- Sometimes found with a surrounding PAM
- Dilated feeder vessels

Ancillary Testing

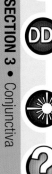

- Excisional biopsy
- Ocular and orbital ultrasound or MRI

Differential Diagnosis

- PAM
- Nevus
- Ocular melanosis

Treatment

- **Varies with extent of lesion:**
  - excisional biopsy and cryotherapy • enucleation • orbital exenteration

Prognosis

- Thickness is most important prognostic factor
- Represent a sight- and life-threatening condition
- Difficult to treat
- Can have local recurrence and distant metastasis (regional lymph nodes, brain, lungs, and liver are most common sites)
- Mortality rate at 10 years' follow-up is around 13%
- Clinician must examine palpebral conjunctiva in all visits after excision to look for recurrence

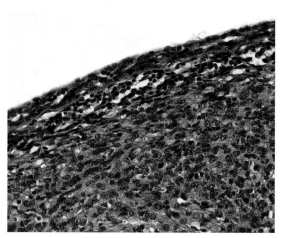

Fig. 3.76 Conjunctival melanoma composed of atypical melanoacytic epitheliod cells with large nuclei and prominent nucleoli. Hematoxylin and eosin, ×400. (Courtesy of Bruno F. Fernandes, MD, and Miguel N. Burnier Jr., MD, PhD.)

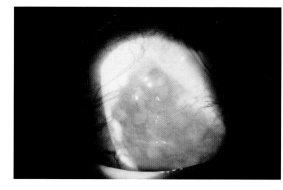

Fig. 3.77 Conjunctival melanoma: pigmented lesion with irregular surface, neovascularization, and ill-defined borders.

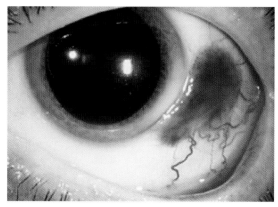

Fig. 3.78 Melanoma on temporal bulbar conjunctiva (limbus is also involved). Note engorged vessels and relatively well-defined margins.

Lymphoid Tumors

Key Facts

- Can be isolated or an ocular manifestation of systemic disease
- Most commonly B-cell lymphoma (non-Hodgkin type)
- Insidious process
- Bilateral disease in ≤38% of cases
- Usually found in the fornices and asymptomatic

Clinical Findings

- Diffuse lesion
- Slightly elevated pink or salmon-colored mass
- Lack of apparent feeder vessels
- Freely movable

Ancillary Testing

- Incisional biopsy
- Complete systemic evaluation

Differential Diagnosis

- Hematic cyst
- Lymphangioma
- Lipoma
- Myxoma

Treatment

- Chemotherapy if systemic disease
- External beam irradiation if localized disease

Prognosis

- Prognostic factors are extent and location of disease
- Development of lymphoma occurs in 30–70% of patients in 10 years

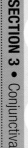

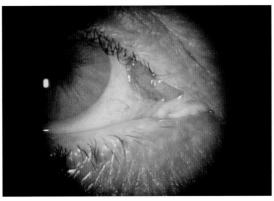

Fig. 3.79 Large and diffuse lesion on superior temporal conjunctiva.

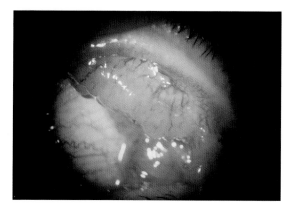

Fig. 3.80 Closer view of the patient in Fig. 3.79. Note salmon color, chemosis, and undefined margins.

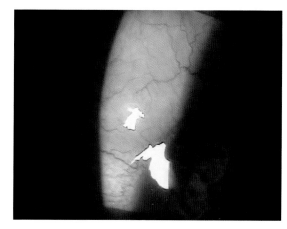

Fig. 3.81 Salmon-colored lymphoid hyperplasia on superior limbus.

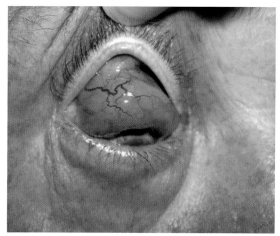

Fig. 3.82 Conjunctival lymphoma. A large fleshy salmon-colored lesion at the superior fornix. (Courtesy of Bruno F. Fernandes, MD.)

Limbal Dermoid

Key Facts
- Congenital lesion, tends to grow with patient
- Occasionally associated with lid colobomas
- Often associated with Goldenhar syndrome
- Can extend to central cornea

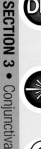

Clinical Findings
- Solid yellow-white mass
- Most commonly found at inferotemporal limbus
- Fine white hairs on tumor's surface

Ancillary Testing
- Evaluate patient for other systemic abnormalities
- Excisional biopsy (can be definitive treatment)

Differential Diagnosis
- Dermolipoma
- Epibulbar osseous choristoma
- Lacrimal gland choristoma
- Goldenhar syndrome

Treatment
- Observation if small asymptomatic lesion
- Excisional biopsy (may penetrate eye wall)
- If involves central cornea, a penetrating keratoplasty may be needed

Prognosis
- Can induce vision loss from corneal astigmatism
- Amblyopia can be a problem, depending on age of onset

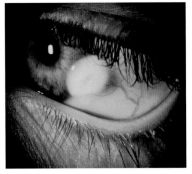

Fig. 3.83 Elevated, white, well-defined limbal dermoid at the inferotemporal limbus.

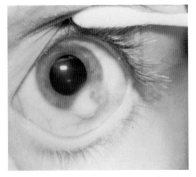

Fig. 3.84 Elevated, white, well-defined limbal dermoid at the inferotemporal limbus.

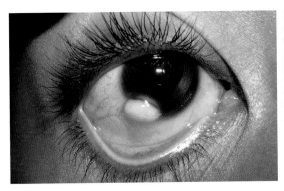

Fig. 3.85 Limbal dermoid: a whitish, well-circumscribed nodule at the inferotemporal limbus. The adjacent corneal epithelium shows an arc-like iron deposition. (Courtesy of Bruno F. Fernandes, MD.)

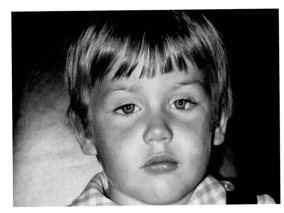

Fig. 3.86 Boy with Goldenhar syndrome. Limbal dermoid on left eye.

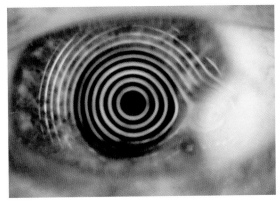

Fig. 3.87 Keratoscopy: irregular astigmatism secondary to limbal dermoid.

Toxic Keratoconjunctivitis

Key Facts

- Caused by chemical trauma
- Patients with dry eyes are particularly at risk
- **Most common causes:**
  - antivirals • antibiotics • glaucoma medications • preservatives

Clinical Findings

- Punctate keratopathy or coarse focal keratopathy
- Pseudodendrites or filamentary keratopathy
- Persistent epithelial defect or geographic ulcers
- Drug deposition
- Papillary, follicular, or mixed conjunctivitis
- Conjunctival scarring or erosions
- Punctal stenosis

Ancillary Testing

- Corneal and conjunctival staining with fluorescein and rose bengal
- Conjunctival scrapings

Differential Diagnosis

- Factitious disease (intentional disease production by patient)
- Allergic conjunctivitis
- Ocular cicatricial pemphigoid or pseudopemphigoid

Treatment

- Drug withdrawal or substitution of non-preserved and less toxic preparations
- Non-preserved artificial tears

Prognosis

- Time taken for improvement and resolution of drug reactions may be prolonged
- Usually non–sight-threatening

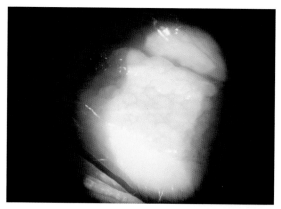

Fig. 3.88 Toxic reaction to topical atropine: chemosis and mixed papillary and follicular reaction on inferior tarsal conjunctiva.

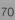

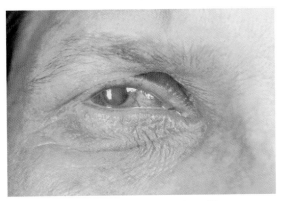

Fig. 3.89 Toxic reaction to topical atropine: diffuse hyperemia, chemosis, and discharge.

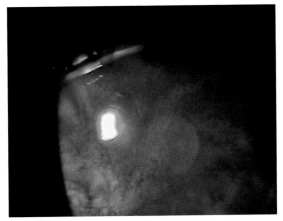

Fig. 3.90 Toxic reaction to topical antiviral medication: superficial punctate keratitis, irregular epithelium, and fluorescein staining.

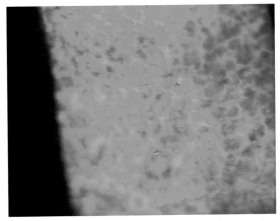

Fig. 3.91 Follicular reaction on the inferior tarsal conjunctiva of the same patient as in Fig. 3.90.

Pingueculae

Key Facts

- Usually bilateral and asymptomatic
- Prevalence increases with age
- Elastotic degeneration of substantia propria (no elastic tissue)
- Predisposing factors thought to be dust and solar exposure
- Can be inflamed and cause ocular irritative symptoms

Clinical Findings

- Elevated white-yellow lesion in interpalpebral conjunctiva
- Lesion does not invade cornea
- Slightly elevated lesion with few or no vessels

Ancillary Testing

- Clinical diagnosis

Differential Diagnosis

- Pterygium
- Conjunctival tumors
- Bitot spot (vitamin A deficiency)

Treatment

- Usually not required
- Typically not recommended merely for cosmetic reasons—risk of recurrence is high
- **When inflamed:** artificial tears, topical non-steroidal anti-inflammatory drugs or steroids
- Surgical excision for recurrent or chronic inflammation

Prognosis

- Non–sight-threatening condition
- Rarely can cause contact lens intolerance
- Surgical excision may result in severe recurrence or progression to pterygium
- Ultraviolet protection can prevent its development

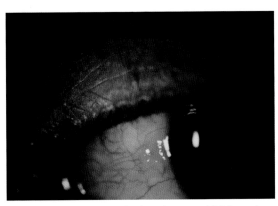

Fig. 3.92 Pinguecula: nasal, triangular area of thickened bulbar conjunctiva in the interpalpebral fissure.

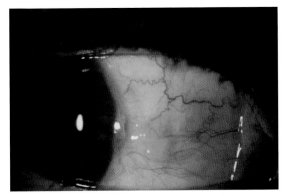

Fig. 3.93 Yellow fleshy appearance of a pinguecula in an 80-year-old patient.

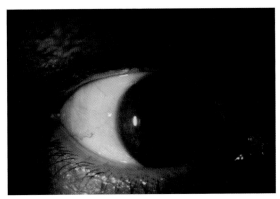

Fig. 3.94 Temporal pinguecula in the same eye of the same patient as in Fig. 3.93.

Pterygium

Key Facts

- Triangular fibrovascular tissue extending from conjunctiva on to cornea
- Males affected more than females
- Most commonly found in patients who live in equatorial regions of the world
- Nasal location more than temporal
- May be exacerbated by keratoconjunctivitis sicca and trauma
- Slowly progressive lesion
- Elastotic degeneration

Clinical Findings

- Slowly progresses centrally ("invades the cornea" may imply that it grows downward through the stroma)
- Destroys Bowman's membrane
- Induces astigmatism and may cause decreased vision
- If it has an iron line at leading edge (Stocker line), more likely to have stopped growing
- Progressive astigmatism

Ancillary Testing

- Assess dry eye status of patient (Schirmer testing; fluorescein, rose bengal, or lissamine green staining)
- Keratometry or corneal topography
- Serial refractions

Differential Diagnosis

- Oblique pterygium
- Terrien marginal degeneration
- Ocular cicatricial pemphigoid
- Chemical burn
- Resolved marginal keratitis
- Squamous cell carcinoma
- Conjunctival intraepithelial neoplasia
- Focal limbal stem cell deficiency

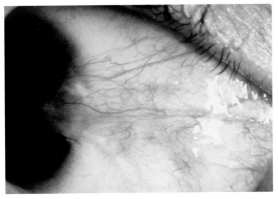

Fig. 3.95 Primary nasal pterygium. Note fibrovascular tissue invading the cornea.

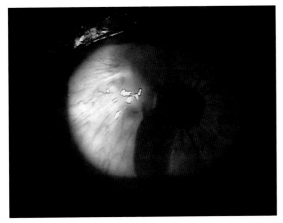

Fig. 3.96 Nasal primary pterygium.

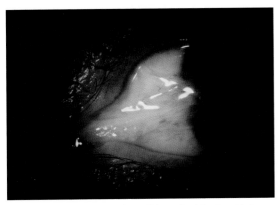

Fig. 3.97 Recurrent pterygium. This patient had restriction of lateral gaze.

Treatment

- Topical lubrication
- Consider punctal occlusion
- **Excision for:**
  - chronic inflammation • contact lens intolerance • vision loss from progressive astigmatism • occlusion of pupil
- Simple excision alone carries a high recurrence rate
- Recurrence rate reduced by conjunctival autograft or amniotic membrane transplantation
- Mitomycin-C
- Fibrin tissue glue

Prognosis

- Good—rare malignant potential
- Without treatment, may extend across cornea and impair vision
- **Recurrence risk depends on:**
  - method of excision • patient longevity • continued ultraviolet exposure

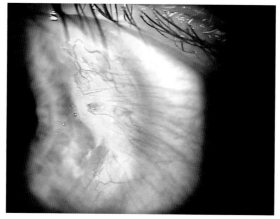

Fig. 3.98 Initial recurrence after pterygium removal.

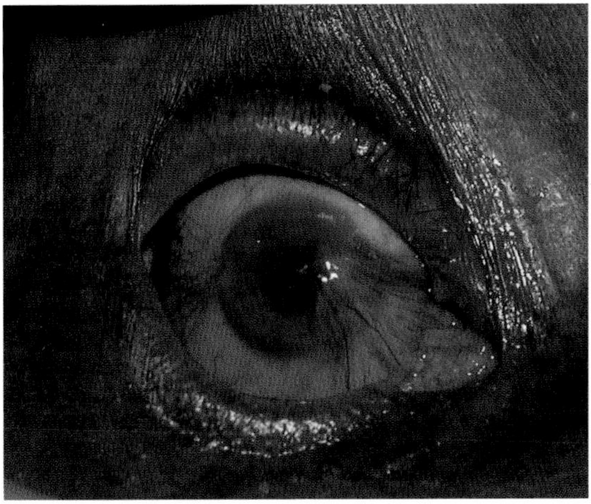

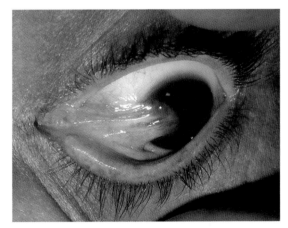

Fig. 3.99 Advanced primary nasal pterygium. (Courtesy of Bruno F. Fernandes, MD.)

Fig. 3.100 Recurrent nasal pterygium. The caruncle is dragged nasally by the fibrovascular tissue. (Courtesy of Bruno F. Fernandes, MD.)

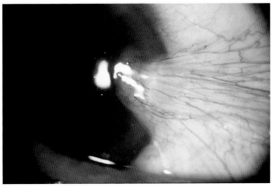

Fig. 3.101 Primary pterygium.

Conjunctivochalasis

Key Facts

- Frequently seen in the elderly
- Can cause ocular irritation and exacerbate dry eye
- May be associated with local inflammation and/or lymphatic dilation
- Usually bilateral

Clinical Findings

- Redundant conjunctiva, usually in the lower bulbar region (may prolapse over lid margin)
- Swollen puncta
- Anterior migration of mucocutaneous junction
- Subconjunctival hemorrhage

Ancillary Testing

- Clinical diagnosis
- Assess dry eye state (Schirmer test, tear break-up time, dye staining)

Differential Diagnosis

- Dry eye
- Conjunctival tumors
- Trichiasis, entropion, or ectropion

Treatment

- Surgical crescent excision (conjunctivoplasty)
- Amniotic membrane transplantation

Prognosis

- Good—low recurrence rate after excision
- Non–sight-threatening condition

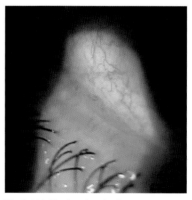

Fig. 3.102 Redundant bulbar conjunctiva; this tends to become more visible on inferior bulbar conjunctiva, folding over the lid margin. There is an association with keratoconjunctivitis sicca.

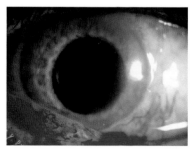

Fig. 3.103 Redundant conjunctiva in the lower temporal quadrant with rose bengal staining. (Courtesy of Carlos Eduardo B. Souza, MD.)

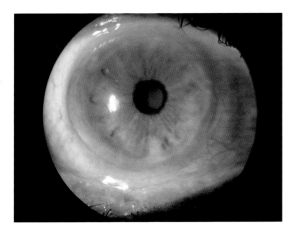

Fig. 3.104 Redundant bulbar conjunctiva.

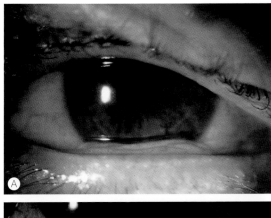

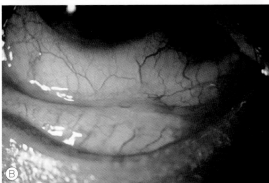

Fig. 3.105 (**A**) A severe case; (**B**) abnormalities on the inferior conjunctiva of the same patient. (Courtesy of Luciene B. de Souza, MD.)

Section 4

Episclera and Sclera

Episcleritis

Key Facts

- More common in young to middle-aged women
- Inflammation confined to superficial episcleral tissue
- Usual complaints include redness and discomfort
- Often idiopathic

Clinical Findings

- Engorgement of superficial episcleral plexus (red or salmon hue)
- Radial configuration of superficial episcleral vessels is preserved
- May be diffuse or associated with nodules
- Rarely associated with systemic rheumatologic disease
- Painless with direct pressure

Ancillary Testing

- Slit-lamp examination with red-free light
- **Topical phenylephrine (2.5–10%) or adrenaline (epinephrine; 1 : 1.000):**
  - Provides blanching of superficial vessels
  - If vessels do not blanch, the vessels are deeper than episcleral and the diagnosis of scleritis must be considered
- Ultrasound biomicroscopy

Differential Diagnosis

- Scleritis
- Conjunctival tumors
- Conjunctivitis
- Chemical burns
- Pingueculitis

Treatment

- Artificial tears
- Topic non-steroidal anti-inflammatory drugs or corticosteroids

Prognosis

- Self-limited condition
- Recurrences can occur
- Non–vision-threatening disease
- Few patients can progress to scleritis

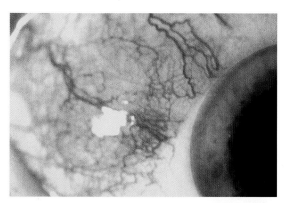

Fig. 4.1 Anterior nodular episcleritis: superficial inflammation without associated symptoms.

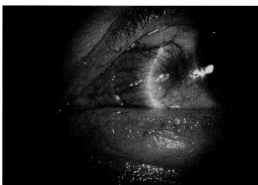

Fig. 4.2 Anterior nodular episcleritis: intense episcleral inflammation. The patient complained only of foreign body sensation.

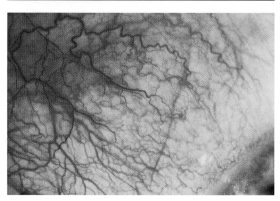

Fig. 4.3 Diffuse episcleritis: the radial configuration of the vessels is preserved.

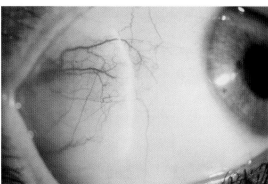

Fig. 4.4 Localized engorgement of the superficial episcleral plexus: no associated symptoms or systemic disease.

Anterior Diffuse Scleritis

Key Facts

- Most common form of scleritis
- Typically a painful process
- Associated with an underlying autoimmune systemic disorder in about half of cases
- More common in women

Clinical Findings

- Diffuse anterior scleral edema
- Dilation of deep episcleral vascular plexus
- Scleral color turns to violet, blue, rosaceous, or salmon hue
- High IOP if involvement of trabecular meshwork

Ancillary Testing

- Complete systemic evaluation to diagnose suspicious underlying disease
- Ocular ultrasonography to evaluate presence of posterior segment findings (e.g. masses and hemorrhage)

Differential Diagnosis

- Migraine
- Giant cell arteritis
- Drug-induced scleritis
- Infectious scleritis
- Iritis
- Episcleritis

Treatment

- Oral non-steroidal anti-inflammatory drugs
- Oral corticosteroids
- Immunosuppressive drugs (depending on associated disease)

Prognosis

- Considered the most benign type of scleritis
- May progress to necrosis
- Vision loss is uncommon but can occur

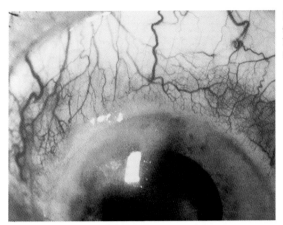

Fig. 4.5 Anterior diffuse sclerokeratitis: the hallmark symptom is pain.

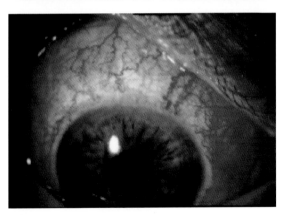

Fig. 4.6 Engorged vessels, with deep scleral inflammation. The sclera has a violet hue.

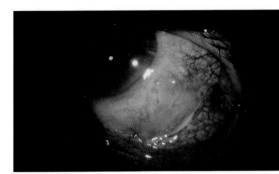

Fig. 4.7 Diffuse scleral hyperemia and dilated vascular plexus. (Courtesy of Luciene B. Souza, MD.)

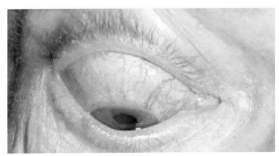

Fig. 4.8 Same patient as in Fig. 4.7. Direct pressure incites extreme discomfort and pain. (Courtesy of Luciene B. Souza, MD.)

Anterior Nodular Scleritis

Key Facts
- Typically a painful process
- Single or multiple nodules
- Associated autoimmune systemic disorder is found in ≤50% of patients
- More common in women

Clinical Findings
- Firm and immobile painful scleral nodule(s)
- Localized areas of scleral edema
- Nodules elevate conjunctival, episcleral, and scleral plexus

Ancillary Testing
- Complete systemic evaluation to diagnose underlying autoimmune disease
- Ultrasonography to evaluate presence of posterior segment findings (e.g. masses and hemorrhage)

Differential Diagnosis
- Infectious scleritis
- Drug-induced scleritis
- Iritis
- Episcleritis

Treatment
- Oral non-steroidal anti-inflammatory drugs
- Oral corticosteroids
- Immunosuppressive drugs (depending on associated disease)

Prognosis
- Depends mostly on associated systemic autoimmune disease, its severity, manifestations, and clinical control
- Permanent vision loss is possible but uncommon

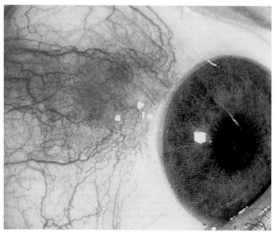

Fig. 4.9 Localized scleral nodule with edema, violet hue, and elevation of conjunctival, episcleral, and scleral vessels.

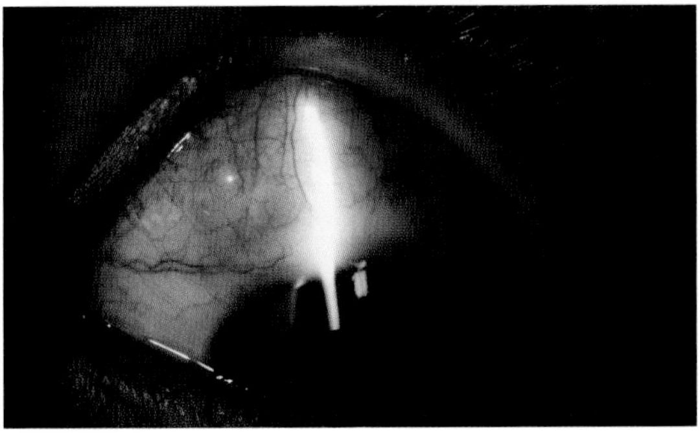

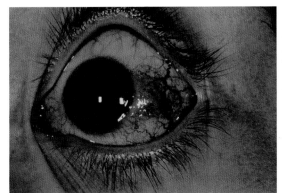

Fig. 4.10 Salmon-colored scleral nodule.

Fig. 4.11 Anterior nodular scleritis. Complete systemic evaluation is warranted to investigate underlying autoimmune disease.

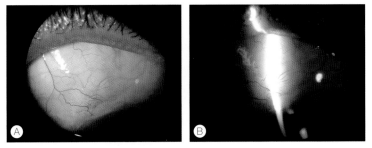

Fig. 4.12 Superior idiopathic anterior nodular scleritis in a 30 year-old female. This case only responded to systemic prednisone.

Necrotizing Scleritis

Key Facts

- Typically excruciatingly painful
- Most severe form of anterior scleritis
- **Often associated with an underlying autoimmune systemic disorder such as:**
    - rheumatoid arthritis • Wegener granulomatosis • relapsing polychondritis
- More common in women

Clinical Findings

- Severe vasculitis
- Areas of capillary non-perfusion, scleral infarction, and necrosis
- Scleral thinning (sometimes underlying uveal tissue becomes visible)
- Spread of process to cornea

Ancillary Testing

- Complete rheumatic evaluation to diagnose underlying autoimmune disease
- Ultrasonography to evaluate for presence of posterior segment findings (e.g. masses and hemorrhage)

Differential Diagnosis

- Infectious scleritis
- Drug-induced scleritis
- Iritis
- Episcleritis

Treatment

- Topical corticosteroids should be avoided—they may contribute to scleral melting
- Oral non-steroidal anti-inflammatory drugs
- Oral corticosteroids
- Immunosuppressive drugs (depending on associated systemic disease)

Prognosis

- Vision loss is common
- Serious threat to eyeball integrity
- Most difficult type of anterior scleritis to treat

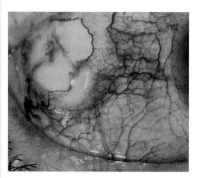

Fig. 4.13 Severe vasculitis, with necrosis of episclera and conjunctiva. Wegener granulomatosis.

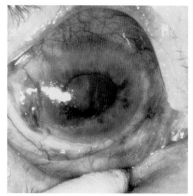

Fig. 4.14 Extensive ischemic and necrotic area, with corneal involvement. The uveal tissue is visible (violet color).

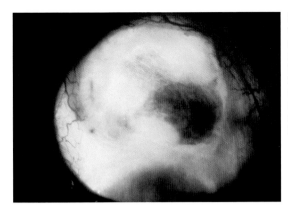

Fig. 4.15 Uveal tissue visible through an area of scleral necrosis and thinning. Prolapsed tissue should be managed very cautiously because of the risk of severe bleeding.

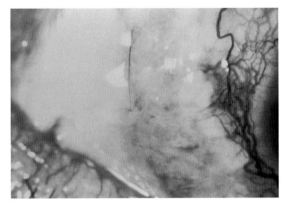

Fig. 4.16 Another example of necrotizing scleritis. Note pale aspect, reflecting scleral, episcleral, and conjunctival non-perfusion and necrosis.

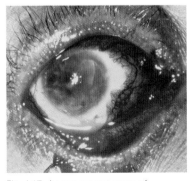

Fig. 4.17 A very severe case of necrotizing scleritis. Guarded prognosis.

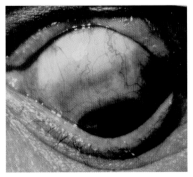

Fig. 4.18 Necrotizing scleritis sequela: extensive area of scleral thinning with visible underlying uveal tissue.

Scleromalacia Perforans

Key Facts
- Obliterative arteritis involving deep episcleral plexus
- Very rare, almost always associated with rheumatoid arthritis
- Typically a painless, asymptomatic process
- More common in elderly women

Clinical Findings
- White, avascular areas
- Scleral thinning with visible underlying uveal tissue

Ancillary Testing
- Complete systemic evaluation
- Ultrasonography

Differential Diagnosis
- Self-inflicted scleritis
- Conjunctival tumors
- Episcleritis

Treatment
- Topical corticosteroids should be avoided—they can contribute to scleral melting
- Oral non-steroidal anti-inflammatory drugs
- Oral corticosteroids
- Immunosuppressive drugs (depending on associated autoimmune disease)

Prognosis
- Associated with increased mortality
- Vision loss can occur
- Ocular perforation is very uncommon

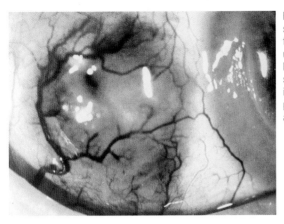

Fig. 4.19 Area of scleral necrosis and thinning, with visible underlying tissue. Note little surrounding inflammation. The patient was asymptomatic.

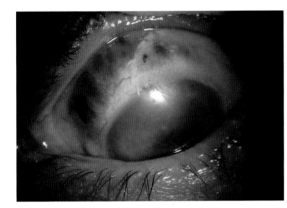

Fig. 4.20 Superior scleral thinning with visible uveal tissue. Minimal inflammation. (Courtesy of the External Eye Disease and Cornea Section, Federal University of Sao Paulo, Brazil.)

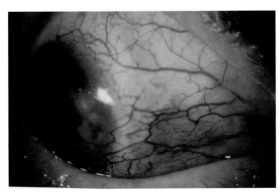

Fig. 4.21 A patient with longstanding rheumatoid arthritis and scleral thinning. (Courtesy of Mario M. Araujo, MD.)

Section 5

Cornea

Epithelial Basement Membrane Dystrophy

Key Facts

- Autosomal dominant, no definitive genetic linkage found
- Widely prevalent disease (most common corneal dystrophy)
- Usual age of diagnosis is 20–40 years
- A small percentage (about 10%) of patients develop recurrent epithelial erosions
- Also known as map–dot–fingerprint or Cogan microcystic epithelial dystrophy
- Corneal periphery is typically unaffected
- Epithelial basement membrane dystrophy is a relative contraindication to LASIK surgery
  - Patients desiring refractive surgery should consider surface ablation instead

Clinical Findings

- **Classic findings (best seen on retroillumination):**
  - maps (large areas of haziness in the basal epithelium, circumscribed by scalloped borders)
  - dots (small round, oval, or comma-shaped opacities)
  - fingerprint (deep epithelial curvilinear and parallel lines)
- Usually the lesions described above follow clear zones and can show negative fluorescein staining (raised areas of epithelium appears dark in the sea of fluorescein)

Ancillary Testing

- Usually a clinical diagnosis (history and slit-lamp examination)
- Histopathologic specimens shows thickened epithelial basement membrane that invaginates into the epithelium in the form of multilaminar sheets of fibrogranular material, and intraepithelial cystic aggregations of degenerating cells underneath an intraepithelial sheet

Differential Diagnosis

- Meesmann epithelial dystrophy
- Reis–Bucklers dystrophy
- Conjunctival intraepithelial neoplasia
- Cornea farinata
- Healing corneal erosion

Treatment

- **Supportive (for recurrent erosions):**
  - topical hypertonic saline • soft bandage contact lens when symptomatic • oral tetracycline antibiotics • topical antibiotic • punctal plug
- Phototherapeutic keratectomy
- Penetrating or lamellar keratoplasty for advanced corneal scarring

Prognosis

- Recurrent erosions can eventually cause irregular astigmatism
- Limbal stem cells harbor the underlying mutation, so recurrence in grafts is not uncommon

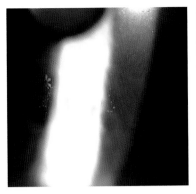

Fig. 5.1 Epithelial cysts (dots). Lesions are surrounded by a clear zone.

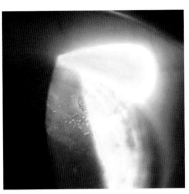

Fig. 5.2 Superficial haziness, with scalloped borders (map) and associated cysts.

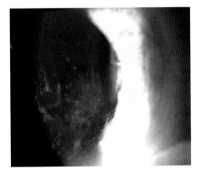

Fig. 5.3 Superficial opacities containing parallel curvilinear lines (fingerprint).

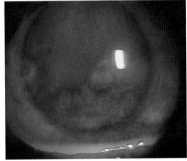

Fig. 5.4 Negative fluorescein staining due to irregular surface.

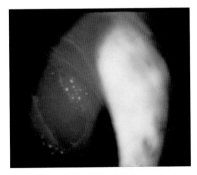

Fig. 5.5 Another example of map lesion and associated cysts.

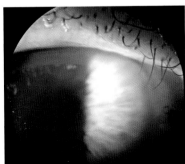

Fig. 5.6 Superficial changes in a patient with recurrent corneal erosions.

Reis–Bücklers Dystrophy

Key Facts

- Bilateral and autosomal dominant disease affecting Bowman's layer
- Mutation in 5q31 in the keratoepithelin gene causes the disease
- Occurs early in childhood, with recurrent episodes of corneal erosion
- Corneal opacification causes decreased vision later in life

Clinical Findings

- Corneal surface appears rough and irregular
- Fine reticular pattern of opacities in Bowman's layer, confined to the central and midperipheral cornea while the extreme periphery is spared

Ancillary Testing

- Usually clinical diagnosis (history and slit lamp examination)
- Consider examining family members
- Histopathologically characterized by pea-like projections from Bowman's layer extending into the epithelium
  - Bowman's layer can be absent in some areas

Differential Diagnosis

- Epithelial basement membrane dystrophy
- Honeycomb dystrophy of Thiel–Behnke
- Grayson–Wilbrandt corneal dystrophy
- Thygeson superficial punctate keratitis

Treatment

- **Supportive (for recurrent erosions):**
  - topical hypertonic saline • soft contact lens • oral tetracycline antibiotics
    - topical antibiotic • punctal plug
- Anterior stromal puncture
- Phototherapeutic keratectomy (PTK)
- Superficial keratectomy
- Lamellar and/or penetrating keratoplasty for advanced corneal scarring

Prognosis

- PTK can be performed for both erosion and visual acuity decrease, with successful results
  - although recurrences are common, PTK can be repeated several times
- Recurrent erosion symptoms gradually subside over second and third decades, with the formation of an anterior stromal haze that compromises vision
- The limbal stem cells harbor the underlying mutation, so recurrence in grafts is common

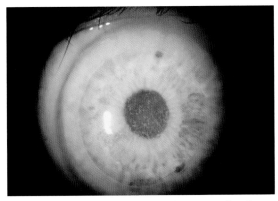

Fig. 5.7 Recurrence of the dystrophy in a corneal graft. Note reticular opacities.

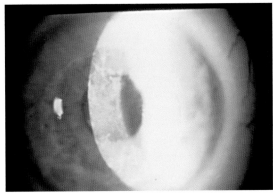

Fig. 5.8 Irregular corneal surface and stromal opacities leading to decreased vision in the patient.

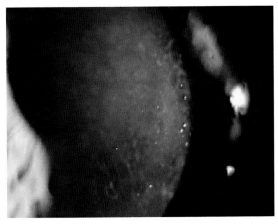

Fig. 5.9 Typical reticular opacities, more numerous in the central cornea. Recurrent erosion episodes lead to scarring and loss of vision.

Granular Dystrophy

Key Facts

- An autosomal dominant disease also known as Groenouw type 1
- Defects in the keratoepithelin gene (Arg555Trp, Arg124H) are responsible
- Slowly progressive, often asymptomatic until later in life
- Corneal erosion episodes occur later in the disease (low incidence)
- Exact nature and source of deposits remain unknown

Clinical Findings

- Sharply demarcated grayish white round or snowflake-like opacities in anterior central stroma
- Lesions centrally located in a random distribution (limbus is typically spared)
- Clear intervening stromal areas
- Surface may stain negatively with fluorescein over superficial lesions

Ancillary Testing

- Usually a clinical diagnosis (history and slit-lamp examination)
- Consider examining family members
- In vivo confocal microscopy
- Histologically characterized by hyaline deposition in stroma and beneath epithelium that stains with Masson trichrome in vitro

Differential Diagnosis

- Avellino corneal dystrophy
- Macular corneal dystrophy

Treatment

- **For recurrent erosions:**
  - topical hypertonic saline • soft contact lens • oral tetracycline antibiotics
    - topical antibiotic • punctal plug
- Phototherapeutic keratectomy (PTK)
- Penetrating or lamellar keratoplasty

Prognosis

- Most patients do not require treatment
- PTK usually achieves successful results, but recurrences tend to be denser and confluent
- Recurrence in grafts may occur as early as 1 year after surgery but usually takes many years

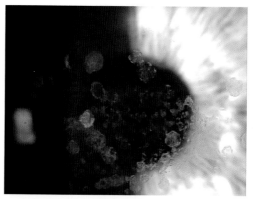

Fig. 5.10 Centrally located snowflake-like opacities with clear intervening zones.

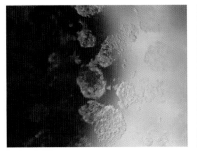

Fig. 5.11 Higher magnification of the image in Fig. 5.10. Random distribution.

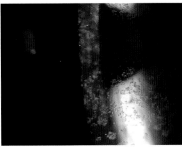

Fig. 5.12 Numerous granular opacities. Patients usually do not experience a dramatic loss of vision.

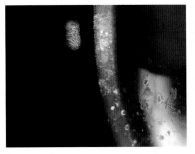

Fig. 5.13 Note central area of haziness due to recurrent erosion.

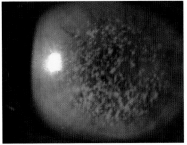

Fig. 5.14 Another example, showing spared peripheral cornea and limbus.

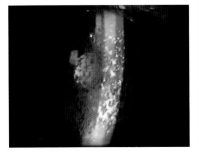

Fig. 5.15 Same patient as in Fig. 5.14: slit view showing stromal location of opacities.

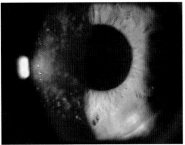

Fig. 5.16 Granular dystrophy 1 month after PTK. At this visit, the patient's best corrected vision was 20/30.

Lattice Dystrophy

Key Facts

- Most common stromal corneal dystrophy
- **Four types have been described:**
  - types 1, 2, and 3a are autosomal dominant, type 3 autosomal recessive
  - type 1 usually develops in teenage years and is associated with recurrent corneal erosions
  - type 2 occurs later in life and primarily involves corneal periphery; relative corneal anesthesia can be found
  - type 3 is characterized by late onset, thicker lattice lines; it is not associated with recurrent erosions
- **Has been associated with the following mutations:**
  - Arg124Cys • Leu518Pro • His626Arg • Asn622His • Leu527Arg

Clinical Findings

- Refractile lattice lines in corneal stroma (best seen on retroillumination), usually centrally located in types 1, 3, and 3a, and peripheral in type 2
- Discrete ovoid or round subepithelial opacities, anterior stromal white dots (early findings)
- Diffuse central anterior stromal haze
- Central corneal sensitivity can be decreased

Ancillary Testing

- Usually a clinical diagnosis (history and slit-lamp examination)
- Consider examining family members
- In vivo confocal microscopy
- Histology shows amyloid deposition, which is positive for Congo red staining seen in anterior and midstroma

Differential Diagnosis

- Avellino dystrophy
- Granular and macular dystrophies

Treatment

- **Recurrent erosions:**
  - patching • hypertonic agents • artificial tears • bandage contact lens • topical antibiotic
- Phototherapeutic keratectomy (PTK) for superficial lesions
- Lamellar and/or penetrating keratoplasty

Prognosis

- Central visual axis is progressively opacified by a stromal haze, with scarring and loss of vision
- The dystrophy is often too deeply located to be completely removed by PTK
- Recurrence in corneal grafts is frequent (more than in granular or macular dystrophies) and can occur as soon as 3 years after surgery
- Secondary glaucoma (due to amyloid deposition in trabecular meshwork) may be present in type 2

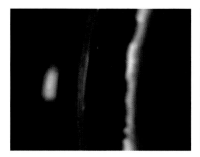

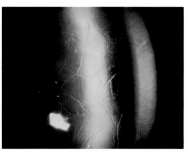

Fig. 5.17 Refractile lattice lines in the corneal stroma.

Fig. 5.18 Retroillumination of lattice lines in detail.

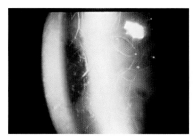

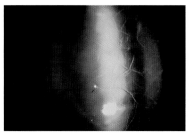

Fig. 5.19 Refractile lattice lines together with stromal haze and subepithelial opacities.

Fig. 5.20 Retroillumination of lattice lines in detail.

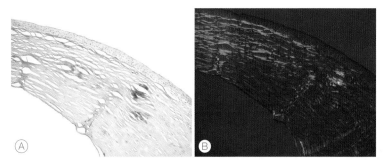

Fig. 5.21 (A) Lattice dystrophy type 1: focal deposits of amyloid are stained in red. Congo red, ×100. (B) Dichroism: the same field viewed with polarized light. The deposits show apple green birefringence. (Courtesy of Bruno F. Fernandes, MD, and Miguel N. Burnier Jr., MD, PhD.)

Avellino Dystrophy

Key Facts

- Combined granular–lattice (variant of granular dystrophy)
- Autosomal dominant condition
- Typically progresses from granular (first) to lattice lesions
- Diagnosis can be confirmed by genetic analysis (replacement of histidine by arginine at codon 124 (R124H) of the BIGH3 gene
- In advanced cases, there is diffuse stromal haze and patients develop recurring erosions
- First described at the University of Minnesota

Clinical Findings

- Anterior, stromal, discrete gray-white granular deposits
- Mid to posterior stromal lattice lesions
- Anterior stromal haze

Ancillary Testing

- Usually clinical diagnosis (history and slit-lamp examination)
- Histology shows granular and fibrillar deposits in anterior stromal layers

Differential Diagnosis

- Lattice dystrophy
- Granular dystrophy
- Reis–Bucklers dystrophy

Treatment

- **For recurrent erosions:**
  - topical hypertonic saline • soft contact lens • oral tetracycline antibiotics • topical antibiotic • punctal plug
- Penetrating or lamellar keratoplasty

Prognosis

- Lesions become more prominent with age, leading to variable loss of vision
- Recurrent corneal erosions can occur
- Recurrence in corneal grafts is not uncommon

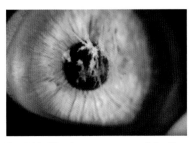

Fig. 5.22 Classic appearance of Avellino dystrophy. (Courtesy of George Rosenwasser, MD.)

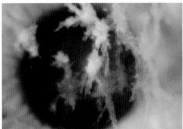

Fig. 5.23 Detailed image from the same patient as Fig. 5.23. (Courtesy of George Rosenwasser, MD.)

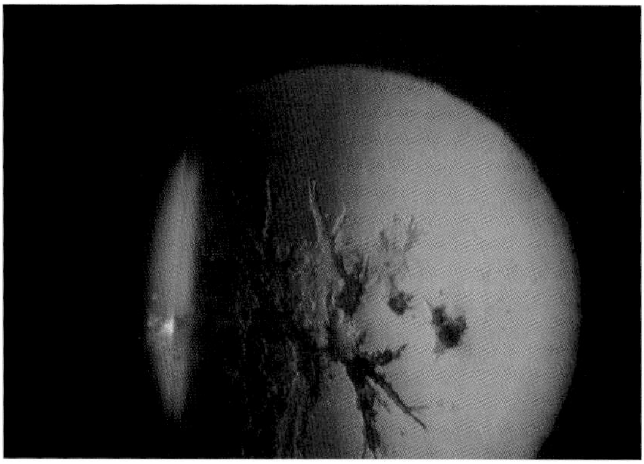

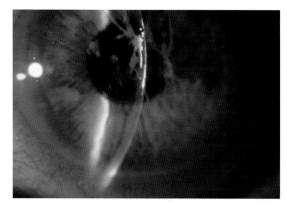

Fig. 5.24 Retroillumination of the same patient as Fig. 5.23. (Courtesy of George Rosenwasser, MD.)

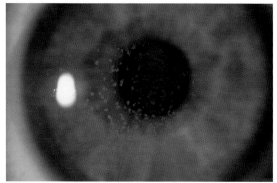

Fig. 5.25 Slit image showing stromal location of the deposits. Same patient as Fig. 5.23. (Courtesy of George Rosenwasser, MD.)

Fig. 5.26 Avellino dystrophy after LASIK. (Courtesy of W. Barry Lee, MD.)

Macular Dystrophy

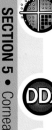

Key Facts

- Autosomal recessive
- Also known as Groenouw type 2
- Least common and most severe of the classic stromal dystrophies
- Chromosomal locus 16q22
- More severe than granular and lattice corneal dystrophies
- May present with recurrent corneal abrasion episodes
- Photophobia, ocular surface discomfort, and progressive loss of vision

Clinical Findings

- Gray-white opacities (intracellular and extracellular deposits within corneal stroma) with indistinct borders and ground glass–like haze in intervening areas
- Lesions can involve full thickness of cornea and be limbus to limbus
- Cornea guttata and reduced central corneal thickness can also be observed

Ancillary Testing

- Pachymetry
- The corneal deposits are glycosaminoglycans (between the stromal lamellae, underneath the epithelium, and within keratocytes and endothelial cells), which stain positively with colloidal iron or Alcian blue in vitro

Differential Diagnosis

- Granular dystrophy
- Reis–Bucklers dystrophy

Treatment

- **For recurrent erosions:**
  - topical hypertonic saline • soft contact lens • oral tetracycline antibiotics • topical antibiotics • punctal plug
- Tinted cosmetic lenses to reduce photophobia
- Phototherapeutic keratectomy (PTK)
- Penetrating or lamellar keratoplasty

Prognosis

- PTK seems to eliminate recurrent erosions and improve vision by ablating opacities in cases of anterior macular dystrophy
- The usual evolution is one of progressive visual impairment, starting to be severe by the third decade and requiring penetrating or lamellar keratoplasty
- Recurrences in corneal grafts are not common, but when occur have the same pattern as the primary disorder
- Size of the graft seems to be inversely related to recurrence (with large graft, low recurrence but increased risk of rejection)

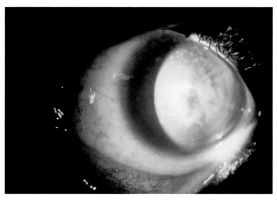

Fig. 5.27 Gray-white opacities with indistinct borders.

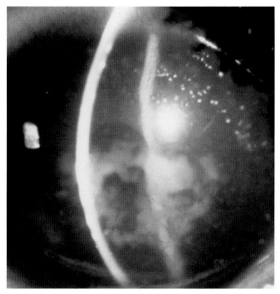

Fig. 5.28 Gray-white opacities with indistinct borders and ground glass-like Laze in the intervening areas.

Schnyder Crystalline Dystrophy

Key Facts

- Autosomal dominant, rare disease
- Chromosomal locus 1p34.1–p36
- Onset early in life
- Corneal erosions are rare
- No regression of lesions has been reported
- Appears to be an imbalance of lipid and cholesterol transport or metabolism
- Variety of symmetric, bilateral corneal lesions are seen

Clinical Findings

- Polychromatic fine crystals can be seen in disciform, geographic, or annular patterns
- Usually, lesions seen in the anterior corneal stroma
  - They occasionally extend into deeper stromal layers
- Intervening stromal areas are usually clear but can show small punctate opacities
- Arcus senilis can be found in peripheral cornea
- Epithelium and corneal sensitivity are normal

Ancillary Testing

- Usually clinical diagnosis (history and slit lamp)
- **In vivo confocal microscopy:** lesions consist of cholesterol crystals and lipid and neutral globular fat deposition
- Evaluate blood levels of cholesterol, triglyceride, and lipoproteins

Differential Diagnosis

- Bietti peripheral crystalline dystrophy
- Cystinosis
- Dysproteinemias (multiple myeloma, Waldenstrom macroglobulinemia, Hodgkin disease)

Treatment

- Lamellar or penetrating grafts may be needed
- Phototherapeutic keratectomy for treating the anterior stromal opacities is still experimental

Prognosis

- Vision is usually not significantly affected, and the disease infrequently progresses
- If penetrating keratoplasty is needed, cholesterol crystals can recur

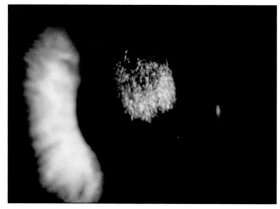

Fig. 5.29 Centrally located lesion with disciform pattern. Intervening stromal areas are clear. Peripheral arcus senilis is noted.

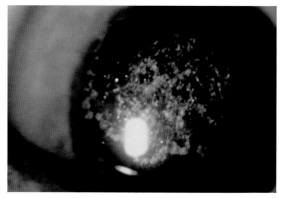

Fig. 5.30 Geographic pattern. Polychromatic fine crystals with intervening small punctate opacities.

Posterior Polymorphous Dystrophy

Key Facts

- Bilateral autosomal dominant posterior membrane dystrophy, highly variable expressivity
- Typically occurs in second or third decade
- Usually asymptomatic, tends to be slowly progressive or non-progressive
- Epithelial characteristics such as desmosomes, tonofilaments, and microvilli are seen on corneal endothelium
- The abnormal cells retain ability to divide and can extend to the trabecular meshwork

Clinical Findings

- Nodular grouped vesicular and blister-like lesions on endothelial surface
- Band-like structures ("railroad tracks"—clinically similar to Haab striae)
- Multilayered endothelium with thickened and multilaminar Descemet's membrane
- Corneal edema in more severe cases
- Iridocorneal adhesions, corectopia, and iris atrophy may occur but are rare
- Corneal epithelium and stroma show no remarkable features

Ancillary Testing

- Specular microscopy
- In vivo confocal microscopy

Differential Diagnosis

- Iridocorneal endothelial syndrome
- Congenital hereditary endothelial dystrophy
- Posterior corneal vesicle syndrome
- Metabolic disease

Treatment

- Control IOP
- Penetrating or endothelial keratoplasty (rarely required)

Prognosis

- The overwhelming majority of patients remain asymptomatic and stable
- The prognosis of graft is strongly related to the presence of anterior synechiae, as well as elevated IOP
- Recurrences after transplantation are described
- Glaucoma and keratoconus have been described in association with this disease

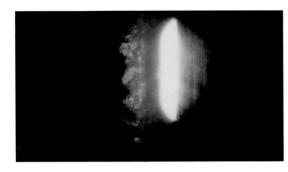

Fig. 5.31 Band-like structures visible on specular reflection. Note irregular endothelial surface.

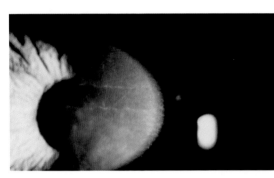

Fig. 5.32 Band-like structures. Differential diagnosis include forceps trauma and Haab striae.

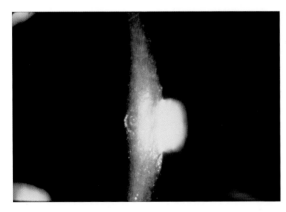

Fig. 5.33 Vesicular (blister-like) lesion on corneal endothelium.

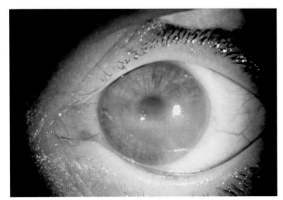

Fig. 5.34 Severe case with corneal edema and epithelial bullae.

Fuchs Dystrophy

Key Facts

- Variable autosomal dominant transmission; may be sporadic. First described in 1910
- Usually manifests after the fourth decade and is a progressive dystrophy
- Females are more affected, and develop corneal guttae 2.5 times more frequently than in males, progressing to corneal edema 5.7 times more often than in males
- Pleomorphic dysfunctional endothelium and an abnormal and thickened basement membrane
- Vision typically worse in the morning and becomes better during the day (due to corneal dehydration)
- Called endothelial dystrophy if guttae without edema
- Called Fuchs dystrophy if guttae in presence of edema

Clinical Findings

- Corneal guttae (hyaline excrescences on Descemet's membrane) is the earliest sign
- Guttae coalesce, creating a beaten metal appearance of the endothelium
- Endothelial polymegathism and pleomorphism
- Overall reduction in endothelial cell density
- Stromal edema, epithelial bullae, and subepithelial fibrosis in advanced cases

Ancillary Testing

- Specular microscopy
- Pachymetry
- In vivo confocal microscopy
- B scan to evaluate posterior segment when cloudy cornea

Differential Diagnosis

- Posterior polymorphous dystrophy
- Iridocorneal endothelial syndrome
- Interstitial keratitis
- Herpes simplex keratitis

Treatment

- Topical hyperosmotic agents, dehydration of the cornea by a blow dryer, reduction of IOP
- Bandage contact lens for recurrent erosion caused by epithelial bullae
- Penetrating or endothelial keratoplasty

Prognosis

- Cataract surgery may accelerate endothelial cell loss, thus worsening corneal edema in patients with otherwise mild disease
  - This depends on each case and surgeon—waiting for the cataract to become dense can also be bad
- The prognosis for penetrating corneal grafts is good (80–90% of clear grafts in 5 years)
- Association with glaucoma is controversial
- The incidence of cataract after penetrating keratoplasty is high
  - surgery carries a good prognosis when performed by experienced surgeons

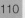

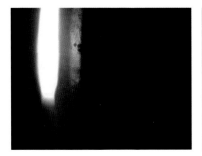

Fig. 5.35 Slit-lamp specular reflex showing corneal guttae.

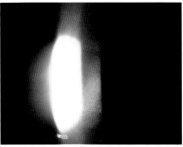

Fig. 5.36 Normal slit-lamp specular reflex in a healthy patient: uniform shape and distribution of endothelial cells.

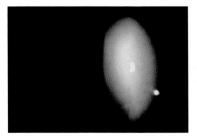

Fig. 5.37 Red reflex: corneal guttae and endothelial abnormalities.

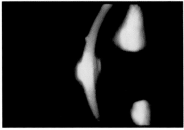

Fig. 5.38 Beaten bronze appearance of the endothelium.

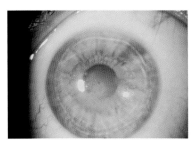

Fig. 5.39 Advanced case of Fuchs dystrophy. Diffuse corneal edema and epithelial bullae.

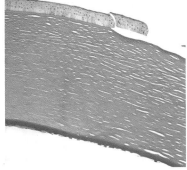

Fig. 5.40 Fuchs endothelial dystrophy: sparse endothelial cells and diffuse and irregular thickening of Descemet's membrane, with wart-like excrescences. An epithelial edema with bullae formation is also seen. Periodic acid Schiff, ×100. (Courtesy of Bruno F. Fernandes, MD, and Miguel N. Burnier Jr., MD, PhD.)

Iridocorneal Endothelial Syndrome

Key Facts

- Non-familial unilateral sporadic disorder (some case reports in the literature of bilateral involvement)
- More common in women (30–50 years old)
- **Diagnosis based on main clinical features:**
  - corneal endothelial abnormalities • iris changes • peripheral anterior synechiae
- **Three different clinical entities described:**
  1. Essential (progressive) iris atrophy
  2. Chandler syndrome
  3. Cogan–Reese syndrome (iris nevus)
- Endothelial cells are diminished in number and display epithelial features (e.g. microvilli, cytoplasmatic tonofilaments, and desmosomal junctions)

Clinical Findings

- Hammered silver appearance of corneal endothelium
- Peripheral anterior synechiae (leading to secondary glaucoma)
- **Iris nevus (Cogan–Reese) syndrome:**
  - nodular pigmented elevations on the iris, no or minimal endothelial changes
- **Chandler syndrome:**
  - corneal endothelial changes predominate
- **Essential (progressive) iris atrophy:**
  - iris atrophy; iris hole formation, corectopia
- Pupil eccentricity is usually found in the direction of the most prominent synechiae
- Stromal and/or epithelial edema
- Band keratopathy may develop in advanced cases

Ancillary Testing

- Specular microscopy
- In vivo confocal microscopy

Differential Diagnosis

- Posterior polymorphous or Fuchs dystrophy
- Iridoschisis and other iris abnormalities (e.g. trauma, uveitis)
- Axenfeld–Rieger syndrome

Treatment

- Topical IOP-lowering agents; glaucoma surgery is often needed
- Penetrating keratoplasty occasionally required (medical therapy is of limited value)

Prognosis

- Progressive disorder, associated with glaucoma in a high number of patients
- Penetrating keratoplasty has a favorable prognosis in most eyes, with good IOP control
  - Essential iris atrophy has the more guarded, and Chandler syndrome the best, prognosis

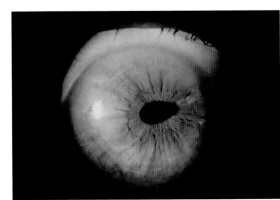

Fig. 5.41 Corectopia in iridocorneal endothelial syndrome: pupil eccentricity in the direction of peripheral anterior synechiae.

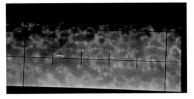

Fig. 5.42 Chandler syndrome: abnormal endothelium, with iridocorneal endothelial syndrome cells.

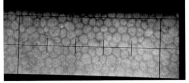

Fig. 5.43 The fellow eye has no alterations—iridocorneal endothelial syndrome is a sporadic, unilateral disease.

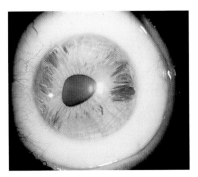

Fig. 5.44 Progressive iris atrophy: corectopia, iris atrophy, and hole formation.

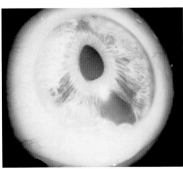

Fig. 5.45 Progressive iris atrophy: corectopia, iris atrophy, and hole formation.

Keratoconus

Key Facts

- Progressive thinning (usually inferior or paracentral) and ectasia of the cornea
- Non-inflammatory process
- No gender or race predominance
- Onset in young adulthood
- Usually bilateral, every corneal layer can be involved
- Transmission pattern can be autosomal dominant or recessive, may be sporadic
- **Association with:**
  - Down syndrome • atopic disease • vernal keratoconjunctivitis • retinitis pigmentosa • Leber congenital amaurosis • aniridia • retinopathy of prematurity • Marfan syndrome • mitral valve prolapse • Ehlers–Danlos syndrome

Clinical Findings

- Conical appearance of the cornea
- Central and inferior stromal thinning (thinnest area is found at apex)
- Retroillumination may show the oil droplet sign, and retinoscopy may show scissoring of the light reflex
- Fleischer ring (iron line surrounding the base of the cone)
- Vogt striae (vertical stress lines in Descemet's membrane)
- Munson sign (angulation of lower lid on down gaze) only in severe cases
- Rizutti sign (sharply focused beam of light near nasal limbus, produced by lateral illumination of the cornea in patients with advanced disease)

Ancillary Testing

- Diagnosis made by clinical presentation
  - Evaluation of red reflex to look for oil droplet sign or scissoring
- Corneal topography
- Ultrasonic or optical pachymetry
- Refraction shows increased myopia with astigmatism
  - As condition progresses, best spectacle-corrected visual acuity may decrease

Differential Diagnosis

- Pellucid marginal degeneration (may exist in tandem with keratoconus)
- Contact lens–induced corneal warpage
- Post-refractive surgery ectasia
- Keratoglobus

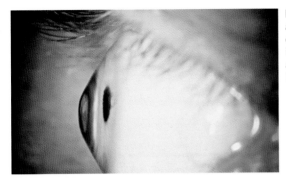

Fig. 5.46 Conical appearance of the cornea (lateral view) in a patient with advanced keratoconus.

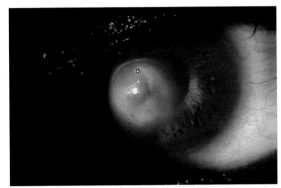

Fig. 5.47 Hydrops usually resolves with clinical treatment but leaves corneal scar that can cause loss of vision and hyperopic shift.

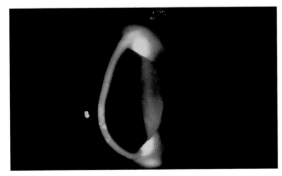

Fig. 5.48 Slit-lamp examination: stromal thinning with thinnest area on cone's apex.

Treatment

- Spectacles or contact lenses (usually rigid gas-permeable lenses give best vision)
- Intracorneal rings (Intacs)
- Corneal transplantation (penetrating or lamellar)
- LASIK must be avoided in these patients—it can contribute to worsening of ectasia

Prognosis

- >80% of patients do not require keratoplasty
- With progressive thinning Descemet's membrane can rupture, causing significant corneal edema (hydrops) with posterior healing and scarring
  - Flattening and improved vision may occur after hydrops resolves
- Keratoplasty has an excellent prognosis, with a success rate of >90% in most series

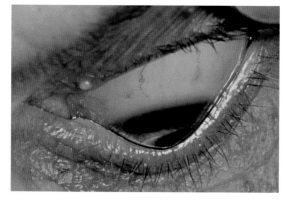

Fig. 5.49 Munson sign in a patient with advanced keratoconus.

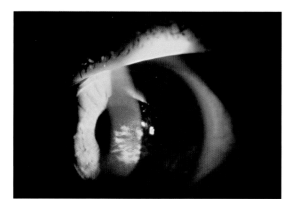

Fig. 5.50 Central corneal scar after hydrops.

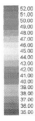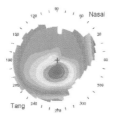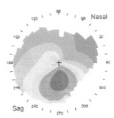

Fig. 5.51 Videokeratography with typical keratoconus pattern. Irregular astigmatism, with steepest area inferiorly.

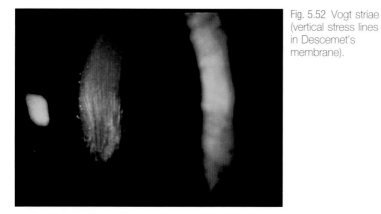

Fig. 5.52 Vogt striae (vertical stress lines in Descemet's membrane).

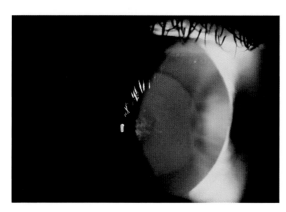

Fig. 5.53 Fleischer ring: iron line surrounding the base of the cone.

Keratoconus (continued)

Pellucid Marginal Degeneration

Key Facts

- Bilateral peripheral corneal thinning and ectatic disorder
- Onset usually at middle age (20–40 years), with no family history
- No race or gender predominance
- Absence of iron deposits, neovascularization, lipid deposition, or epithelial abnormalities

Clinical Findings

- Crescent-shaped band of thinning in inferior portion of cornea (typically spanning from the 4 to 8 o'clock position), with peripheral band of normal cornea
- The protruded area is superior to the thinning band
- Thinned area is clear and about 1–2 mm wide
- Against the rule astigmatism

Ancillary Testing

- Diagnosis made by clinical presentation
- Videokeratography (corneal topography)
- Ultrasonic or optical pachymetry

Differential Diagnosis

- Keratoconus
- Terrien marginal degeneration
- Idiopathic furrow degeneration
- Mooren ulcer

Treatment

- Spectacles or contact lenses (usually rigid gas-permeable lenses give best vision)
- Eccentric lamellar or penetrating keratoplasty for resection of thinned area
- LASIK must be avoided in these patients—it can contribute to worsening of ectasia

Prognosis

- The ectasia can progress over time, leading to hydrops and corneal scarring
- Surgery generally unsatisfactory because the pathology is in the corneal periphery
  - Complications of keratoplasty include irregular astigmatism, neovascularization, and graft rejection

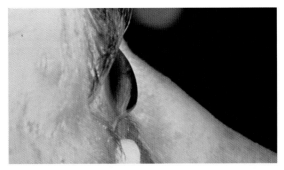

Fig. 5.54 Advanced case: lateral view.

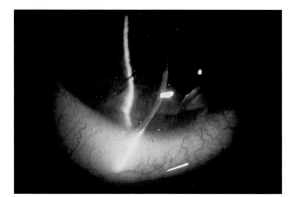

Fig. 5.55 Inferior thinned area with superior protrusion. Note absence of neovascularization or epithelial abnormalities.

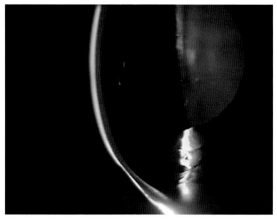

Fig. 5.56 Inferior crescent-shaped band of thinning in the peripheral cornea, with normal thickness cornea on either side.

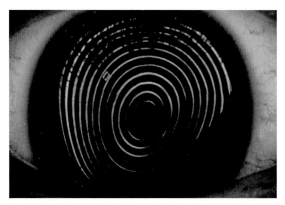

Fig. 5.57 Irregular astigmatism in a patient with pellucid marginal degeneration.

Salzmann Nodular Degeneration

Key Facts

- Occurs typically in eyes with chronic inflammation or dryness
- Unilateral or bilateral
- More common in women, usually asymptomatic (unless the visual axis is affected or astigmatism is induced)
- **Associated with many diseases, such as:**
  - immune stromal keratitis • vernal keratoconjunctivitis • trachoma • herpetic keratitis • keratoconjunctivitis sicca • phlyctenular disease

Clinical Findings

- Single or multiple white, gray-white, or bluish elevated corneal lesions, often annular in location
- Each nodule is separated from other by clear cornea, and iron lines may be present
- More commonly adjacent to an area of corneal scarring, edema, and neovascularization
- Irregular astigmatism

Ancillary Testing

- Usually a clinical diagnosis (history and slit-lamp examination)
- Topography helpful in evaluating level of irregular astigmatism

Differential Diagnosis

- Corneal scar or keloid
- Band keratopathy
- Lipid keratopathy
- Conjunctival intraepithelial neoplasia
- Amyloidosis
- Epithelial basement membrane dystrophy

Treatment

- Lubrication
- Superficial or phototherapeutic keratectomy
- Rigid gas-permeable lenses for visual rehabilitation
- Lamellar or penetrating keratoplasty for severe scarring

Prognosis

- Epithelial erosions may overlie the lesion
- Corneal grafts have an excellent prognosis for survival, but recurrence has been reported

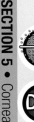

SECTION 5 • Cornea

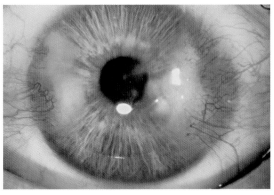

Fig. 5.58 Gray-white elevated Salzmann nodules adjacent to recurrent pterygium.

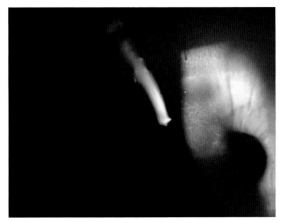

Fig. 5.59 Slit lamp: corneal opacification secondary to Salzmann nodular degeneration.

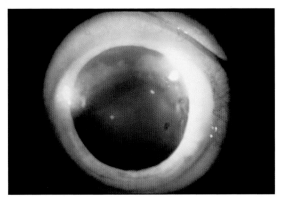

Fig. 5.60 Numerous bluish nodules in an annular pattern. Note that each nodule is separated by a clear space.

Terrien Marginal Degeneration

Key Facts

- Slowly progressive bilateral peripheral corneal inflammatory and degenerative disorder
- Rare disease with unknown etiology
- More common in men (3 : 1 ratio) between 20 and 40 years of age
- Can begin in area of oblique pterygium

Clinical Findings

- Small white opacities in anterior stroma (usually in supranasal peripheral cornea)
- Superficial vascularization from limbal arcades
- Peripheral corneal thinning with an intact epithelium
- Lipid deposits can be seen in the advancing edge
- Against the rule astigmatism

Ancillary Testing

- Corneal topography
- Corneal pachymetry

Differential Diagnosis

- Idiopathic furrow degeneration
- Mooren ulcer
- Corneal dellen
- Pellucid marginal degeneration

Treatment

- No treatment to prevent disease from advancing
- Spectacles or contact lenses (usually rigid gas-permeable lenses give best vision)
- Eccentric lamellar or penetrating keratoplasty for resection of thinned area

Prognosis

- Thinning may progress circumferentially or be stationary
- In most cases, thinning does not progress to perforation
- Surgery generally unsatisfactory, with high postoperative complications (e.g. irregular astigmatism, neovascularization, and graft rejection)

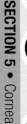

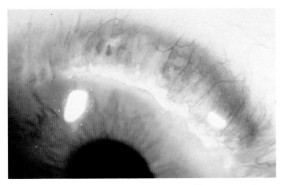

Fig. 5.61 Superior corneal involvement in Terrien marginal degeneration: neovascularization, stromal thinning, and central lipid deposition.

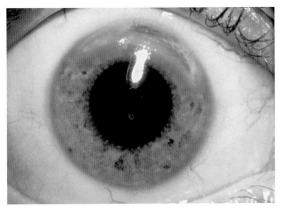

Fig. 5.62 Peripheral corneal thinning. No associated ocular inflammation.

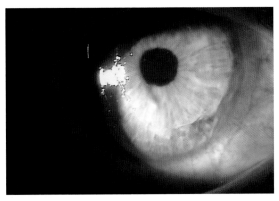

Fig. 5.63 Terrien marginal degeneration beginning in an area of oblique pterygium. Peripheral corneal thinning with intact epithelium.

Cornea Verticillata

Key Facts

- Consists of deposits in the corneal epithelium
- Usually seen as side effect of certain systemic medications or secondary to sphingolipidoses (such as Fabry disease)
- **Related medications include:**
  - amiodarone • tamoxifen • atovaquone • chloroquine • chlorpromazine • indomethacin
- **In Fabry disease (X-linked recessive disease), female carriers can develop these corneal alterations and affected males can present with:**
  - periorbital edema • conjunctival vessel tortuosity and dilation • papilledema • retina edema • optic atrophy • spoke-like posterior cataracts
- Amiodarone, tamoxifen, and chloroquine are reported to be associated with optic neuropathy and maculopathy

Clinical Findings

- Subepithelial or epithelial fine lines that swirl from a point below the center of the cornea and radiate to the periphery in a vortex-like pattern

Ancillary Testing

- Clinical diagnosis (history and slit-lamp examination)

Differential Diagnosis

- Fabry disease
- Multiple sulfatase deficiency
- Generalized gangliosidosis
- Multiple myeloma
- Medication deposit
- Striate melanokeratosis
- Iron depositions
- Anterior crocodile shagreen

Treatment

- Usually no ocular treatment is required

Prognosis

- Usually does not cause visual disturbances (rarely glare and haloes at night)
- Deposits generally reversible with discontinuation of medication
- In Fabry disease, the visual prognosis is excellent and death is usually secondary to renal, cardiac, or cerebrovascular disease

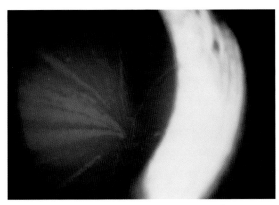

Fig. 5.64 Fabry disease: epithelial lines swirling from a point below the center of the cornea.

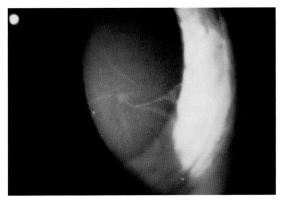

Fig. 5.65 Corneal epithelial deposits in a patient taking amiodarone.

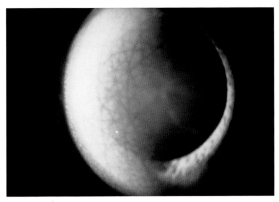

Fig. 5.66 Crocodile shagreen. Corneal degeneration as a differential diagnosis.

Thygeson Superficial Punctate Keratitis

Key Facts

- Uncommon corneal epitheliopathy of unknown etiology
- Chronic condition with spontaneous remissions and transient exacerbations
- Usually bilateral disease
- No race or gender predilection in most reports
- Associated with HLA-DR3
- Usually diagnosed during second or third decade (range 2.5–85 years)
- Healing without corneal scarring, lack of response to antibiotics and antivirals
- Lesions entirely epithelial and do not incite neovascularization

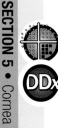

Clinical Findings

- Discrete round or oval grouped punctate intraepithelial deposits, usually in central to paracentral cornea (range 1–50 lesions)
- Each deposit consists of numerous discrete, fine, granular, white to gray dot-like opacities
- Mild epithelial and subepithelial edema
- Lesions slightly elevated during exacerbations
  - Epithelium between lesions is normal • Little or no conjunctival hyperemia

Ancillary Testing

- Clinical diagnosis (history and slit-lamp examination)

Differential Diagnosis

- Staphylococcal inflammatory marginal keratitis
- Seborrheic blepharitis
- Keratoconjunctivitis sicca or exposure keratopathy
- Herpetic keratitis
- Recurrent erosion syndrome
- Keratitis secondary to blepharitis, meibomian gland dysfunction, or contact lenses

Treatment

- Low-dose topical steroids (during exacerbations)
- Topical non-steroidal anti-inflammatory drugs may play a role
- Therapeutic (bandage) contact lenses
- Topical cyclosporin A 2%
- Tinted lenses during exacerbations

Prognosis

- Visual prognosis is good (non–sight-threatening condition)
- Typically the more spots seen, the more symptomatic the patient
- The disease usually has a chronic course and can last more than a decade, but signs and symptoms often resolve spontaneously

Fig. 5.67
Epitheliopathy: discrete, grouped round and oval deposits in central cornea with mild surrounding edema.

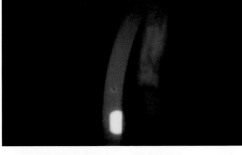

Fig. 5.68 Detail of a single elevated lesion. Negative staining with fluorescein dye.

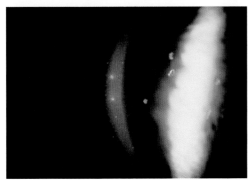

Fig. 5.69 Another example of negative staining. Bilateral disease with no neovascularization or conjunctival injection.

Fig. 5.70 Thygeson superficial punctate keratitis: note that the epithelium between lesions is normal.

Band Keratopathy

Key Facts

- Chronic degenerative condition with calcium deposition at Bowman's membrane, epithelial basement membrane, and anterior corneal stroma
- Typically seen in eyes with chronic inflammation
- Can be associated with systemic diseases

Clinical Findings

- Grayish opacification of cornea, typically beginning in peripheral cornea (at 3 and 9 o'clock positions)
- Most frequently seen in interpalpebral zone, separated from the limbus by a clear area
- Swiss cheese appearance due to scattered holes inside the band, where corneal nerves penetrate through Bowman's layer
- A fibrous pannus may separate the epithelium and Bowman's layer

Ancillary Testing

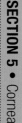

- Clinical diagnosis (history and slit-lamp examination)
- Systemic work-up

Differential Diagnosis

- Arcus senilis
- Limbal girdle of Vogt
- Salzmann nodular degeneration
- Spheroidal degeneration

Treatment

- Ocular lubrication
- Disodium EDTA chelation (0.05 molar concentration)
- Phototherapautic keratectomy with excimer laser
- Lamellar keratoplasty

Prognosis

- Usually asymptomatic unless extends to visual axis
- Generally slow progression (dry eye can exacerbate the disease)
- Accumulation of calcium can disrupt the ocular surface, causing irritation, photophobia, or recurrent erosions
- Recurrences after treatment are somewhat common, especially when underlying causative condition persists

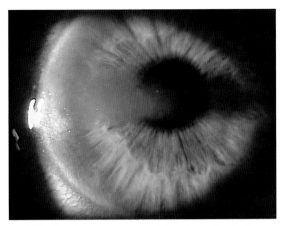

Fig. 5.71 Classic appearance: calcium deposition in the interpalpebral zone.

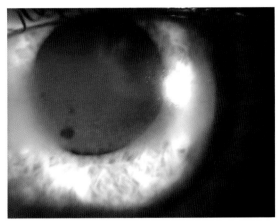

Fig. 5.72 Band keratopathy: note Swiss cheese appearance. Longstanding anterior uveitis.

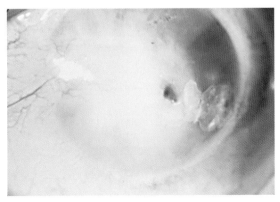

Fig. 5.73 Band keratopathy and neovascularization in a patient with chronic syphilitic interstitial keratitis.

Common Etiologies

- Chronic ocular disease:
  interstitial keratitis
  phthisis
  chronic uveitis
  chronic corneal edema
  chronic keratitis
- Hypercalcemic states
  hyperparathyroidism
  sarcoidosis
  vitamin D toxicity
- Hypophosphatemia
- Intraocular silicone oil
- Chemical exposure in ophthalmic medications
- Keratoconjunctivitis sicca
- Systemic disease
- Primary hereditary band keratopathy
- Idiopathic

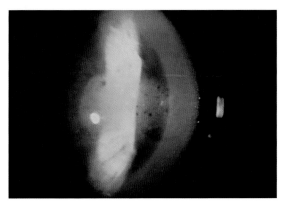

Fig. 5.74 Band keratopathy with a central elevated area. Recurrent erosions can occur.

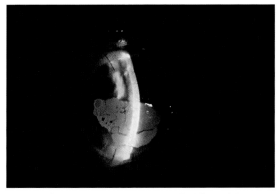

Fig. 5.75 Ciprofloxacin deposit in a graft: differential diagnosis. (Courtesy of Paulo Cesar Fontes, MD.)

Mooren Ulcer

Key Facts

- Chronic, progressive, painful peripheral ulceration of the cornea
- Rare disease of unknown etiology (presumed autoimmune), no definitive association with gender and/or race
- Corneal surgery, infections, and/or accidental injuries have been reported in patients before clinical manifestation of Mooren ulcer, although most cases are idiopathic
- Association with hepatitis C virus infection and helminthiasis has been suggested but not proven
- **Distinct clinical types described:**
  - type 1 (*typical* or *non-progressive*): unilateral in about 75% of cases, seen in older patients, usually responds well to medical therapy
  - type 2 (*progressive* or *malignant*): bilateral in about 75% of patients, most common in younger ages, relentlessly progressive despite any therapy

Clinical Findings

- Gray-white, crescent-shaped peripheral corneal ulcer
- Intense limbal inflammation undermining central edge of ulcer
- Usually no clear zone between ulcer and limbus, progresses centrally and circumferentially
- Melting of anterior one-third to one-half of stromal thickness, with consequent scarring and thinning
- Healing occurs with neovascularization originating from the conjunctiva
- Episcleritis and/or scleritis can be associated, as well as anterior uveitis, cataract, and secondary glaucoma

Ancillary Testing

- Usually a clinical diagnosis (history and slit-lamp examination)
- Systemic work-up to rule out autoimmune or infectious diseases (included hepatitis C and helminthiasis)

Differential Diagnosis

- Systemic malignancies, vasculitis, and collagen diseases (e.g. Wegener granulomatosis, polyarteritis nodosa, and rheumatoid arthritis)
- Terrien marginal degeneration
- Furrow degeneration
- Pellucid marginal degeneration
- Staphylococcal marginal keratitis
- Acne rosacea

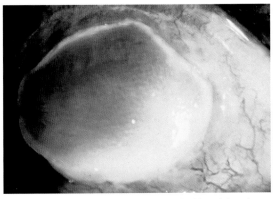

Fig. 5.76 Gray-white, crescent-shaped 360° peripheral ulcer. Limbal inflammation and corneal neovascularization.

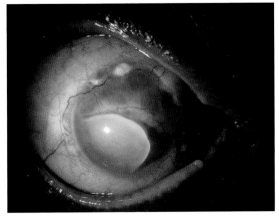

Fig. 5.77 Advanced Mooren ulcer: severe corneal scarring and thinning. (Courtesy of the External Eye Disease and Cornea Section, Federal University of Sao Paulo, Brazil.)

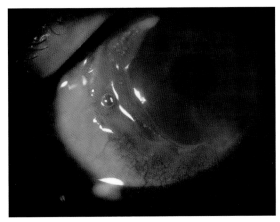

Fig. 5.78 Typical Mooren ulcer: peripheral ulcer, thinning, and inflammation. (Courtesy of Guilherme Rocha, MD.)

Treatment

- Topical steroids (prednisolone 1% every hour) or systemic immunosuppressive agents
- Subcutaneous injections of interferon alfa-2b when associated with hepatitis C infection
- Intravenous humanized lymphocytotoxic monoclonal antibody (Campath-1H)
- Surgical excision of the conjunctiva adjacent to the ulcer
- Lamellar keratectomy, lamellar scleral autograft, multilayered amniotic membrane

Prognosis

- Often progresses to visual loss (caused by irregular astigmatism, direct involvement of visual axis, and/or associated anterior uveitis, cataract, and glaucoma) despite all attempts at management and therapy
- Perforation with minor trauma has been noted in ≤35% of cases
- Attempts at penetrating keratoplasty often associated with recurrence and graft failure

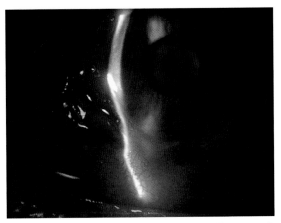

Fig. 5.79 Same patient as Fig. 5.78: slit view. (Courtesy of Guilherme Rocha, MD.)

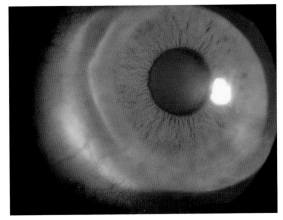

Fig. 5.80 Same patient as in Fig. 5.78 after immunosuppression: healed ulcer. (Courtesy of Guilherme Rocha, MD.)

Peripheral Ulcerative Keratitis

Key Facts

- Acute corneal ulceration, inflammation, or melting
- May be associated with autoimmune or collagen vascular disease
- May be associated with blepharitis or rosacea
- Rapidly progressive
- May cause corneal perforation
- Re-epithelialization required before resolution

Clinical Findings

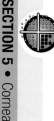

- Peripheral corneal infiltration progressing to ulceration and thinning
- May spread circumferentially
- **May be associated with:**
  - pain • discharge • photophobia • red eye • decreased vision
- Most commonly seen in inferonasal and inferotemporal quadrants • Anterior chamber cell flare • Hypopyon-associated scleritis • Episcleritis • Ancillary injection possible

Ancillary Testing

- Complete examination with attention to lids
- Fluorescein staining of anterior chamber
- **Laboratory tests, including:**
  - complete blood count • erythrocyte sedimentation rate • rheumatoid factor • antinuclear antibody • antineutrophil
- Cytoplasmic antibodies (ANCA)
- Corneal cultures or smears to rule out infectious etiology
- Rheumatology consult for systemic disorders

Differential Diagnosis

- Tuberculosis
- Autoimmune disease
- Rosacea
- *Staphylococcus* marginal blepharitis
- Collagen vascular disease

Treatment

- Topical antibiotics if epithelial defect exists
- Cycloplegic agent if anterior chamber cell and flare exist
- Topical steroids if infectious etiology ruled out
- Lid hygiene and warm compresses for blepharitis
- Oral doxycycline 50–100 mg p.o. q.d. for blepharitis
- Topical lubrication and protective eyewear
- Immunosuppressive agents if autoimmune etiology identified
- Lamellar keratectomy, conjunctival resection may be required

Prognosis

- Good for marginal keratitis secondary to blepharitis
- Underlying etiology must be identified and treated
- Long-term immunomodulation may be required
- Poor if marginal keratolysis due to untreated autoimmune disorders or Mooren ulcer

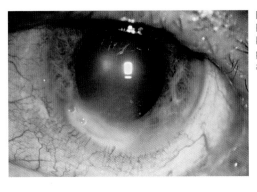

Fig. 5.81 Peripheral ulcerative keratitis: inferior lesion in a patient with rheumatoid arthritis.

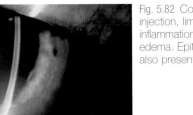

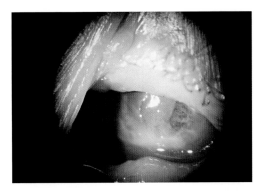

Fig. 5.82 Conjunctival injection, limbal inflammation, and corneal edema. Epithelial defect is also present.

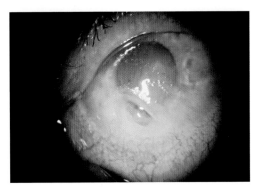

Fig. 5.83 Perforated ulcer in a patient with Wegener granulomatosis. Guarded prognosis.

Fig. 5.84 Another example of perforation in peripheral ulcerative keratitis. This patient had severe keratoconjunctivitis sicca.

Neurotrophic Keratopathy

Key Facts

- Degenerative corneal disease caused by impairment of trigeminal corneal innervation leading to a decrease or absence of corneal sensation and healing impairment
- Cell vitality is compromised by local changes in the level of neuromediators
- **The corneal epithelium is the first target:**
  - decreased overall thickness • cells show intracellular swelling • loss of microvilli • abnormal production of basal lamina

Clinical Findings

- Mackie classification
  Stage 1:
  - punctate keratopathy, epithelial hyperplasia and irregularity • superficial neovascularization and/or scarring • increased viscosity of tear mucus, decreased break-up time • dellen, small facets of drying epithelium (Gaule spots)

  Stage 2:
  - persistent epithelial defect (most frequent in the superior half cornea) with smooth and rolled edges • poorly adherent, opaque, and edematous epithelium surrounding defect • Descemet's folds, stromal swelling, anterior chamber reaction

  Stage 3:
  - stromal lysis, with corneal ulcer that may progress to melting and/or perforation

Ancillary Testing

- Usually a clinical diagnosis (history and slit-lamp examination)
- Cochet–Bonnet aesthesiometer to localize and quantify corneal sensitivity
- Assess ocular surface carefully (break-up time, lissamine green, rose bengal and fluorescein staining, Schirmer test)

Differential Diagnosis

- Infective, toxic, immune corneal ulcers
- Dry eye
- Exposure keratitis
- Topical drug toxicity
- Contact lens abuse
- Persistent central corneal epithelial defect secondary to limbal stem cell deficiency

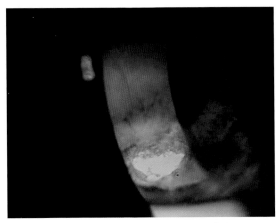

Fig. 5.85 Stage 2 neurotrophic keratopathy: inferior epithelial defect with smooth edges, and surrounding edema.

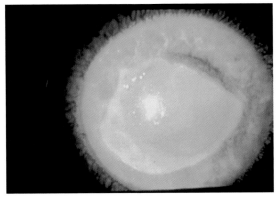

Fig. 5.86 Large neurotrophic ulcer. Note oval shape, rolled edges, and surrounding edema.

Neurotrophic Keratopathy (Continued)

Treatment

- Discontinuation of all topical medications and evaluate side effects of systemic therapies
- Topical preservative-free artificial tears, correct eyelid dysfunction, consider punctal occlusion
- Oral doxycycline, topical medroxyprogesterone, topical autologous serum
- Cyanoacrylate glue, lateral tarsorrhaphy, amniotic membrane transplantation, conjunctival flap
- Lamellar or penetrating keratoplasty in larger defects

Prognosis

- Challenging disease—the more severe the corneal sensory impairment, the higher the probability of disease progression
- Progression of the disease may lead to corneal ulcers, melting, and perforation
- Lamellar or penetrating keratoplasties are high-risk procedures with frequent complications and should be done only with a lateral tarsorrhaphy

Most Common Etiologies

Systemic

- Diabetes • Leprosy • Vitamin A deficiency

Central nervous system

- Neoplasms or aneurysms • Stroke • Surgical injuries

Ocular

- Post herpes infections • Chemical and physical burns • Drug toxicity • Chronic ocular surface disease • Contact lens wear

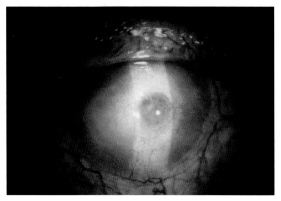

Fig. 5.87 Stage 3 ulcer: perforation after stromal lysis.
(Courtesy of Paulo Cesar Fontes, MD.)

Central Bacterial Ulcer

Key Facts

- Relatively common (estimated incidence of 30 000 cases per year in the USA)
- No specific signs to establish definite bacterial cause
- Most common organisms are *Staphylococcus* species and *Pseudomonas*
- **Known risk factors include:**
  - contact lens wear (most common risk factor in developed nations) • corneal trauma, lagophthalmos, corneal exposure • systemic diseases (e.g. diabetes mellitus) • dry eye, eyelid infection, canaliculitis • chronic use of steroids and/or antibiotics • ocular surface and corneal diseases
- **Few bacteria can directly penetrate corneal epithelium to initiate stromal suppuration:**
  - *Neisseria gonorrhea* • *N. meningitidis* • *Corynebacterium diphtheriae* • *Haemophilus aegyptius* • *Shigella* • *Listeria*

Clinical Findings

- Conjunctival hyperemia, chemosis, purulent secretion
- Suppurative stromal infiltrate, epithelial defect with indistinct edges, edema
- White cell infiltration into surrounding stroma, hypopyon, anterior chamber reaction

Ancillary Testing

- Fluorescein and rose bengal staining of cornea
- **Microbiologic investigation (material obtained by corneal scraping or biopsy):**
  - microscopy (gram stains) • culture (blood agar, chocolate agar, Sabouraud agar, thioglycolate broth); Sabouraud agar is a fungal culture (important to investigate mixed infections), thioglycollate is a liquid media for bacteria and excellent for broad species culture including anaerobes • antimicrobial susceptibility testing

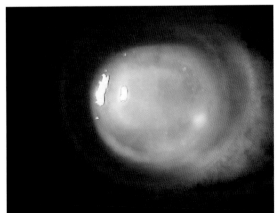

Fig. 5.88
Pseudomonas keratitis in a contact lens wearer. Central ulcer with suppurative stromal inflammation and infiltration into surrounding stroma.

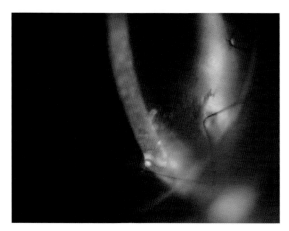

Fig. 5.89 Crystalline infectious keratopathy in a corneal graft. The most common causative organism is *Streptococcus viridans*.

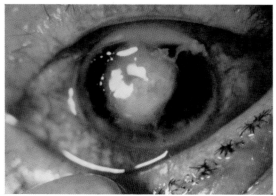

Fig. 5.90 Severe infectious keratitis. Note stromal infiltration and lysis.

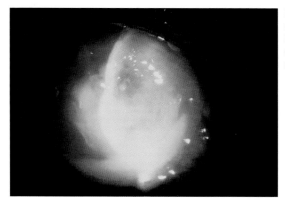

Fig. 5.91 Diffuse corneal infectious keratitis, with anterior chamber reaction and hypopyon.

Differential Diagnosis

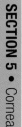

- Non-bacterial corneal pathogens (e.g. *Acanthamoeba* and fungi)
- Herpetic keratitis
- Factitious keratoconjunctivitis
- Chemical, thermal, or mechanical injuries
- *Staphylococcus* marginal keratitis

Treatment

- No single antibiotic is effective against all potential causative organisms
  - Decision on whether or not to use fortified antibiotics should be made according to severity of disease • Close follow-up is warranted (daily visits at beginning of therapy), and modifications in antibiotic therapy should be guided by clinical response (most important) and microbiologic results
- **Severe keratitis (empiric treatment):** topical cefazolin (50 mg/mL) combined with tobramycin (14 mg/mL)
  - First, load the cornea every minute for 15 min to ensure compliance, then hourly for the first 24–36 h • If good clinical response, keep both antibiotics every 3 h until resolution • If poor response, change antibiotics guided by culture and antimicrobial susceptibility testing
- **Less severe keratitis (empiric treatment):** topical fluoroquinolone (gatifloxacin or moxifloxacin) with commercially available concentrations hourly for first 24–36 h, then every 3 h until resolution
- Subconjunctival antibiotic injections may be indicated in special cases
- **Systemic antibiotics indicated when:**
  - severe keratitis with impending perforation • perforated infections with potential for intraocular spread • after perforating injuries to corneosclera • contiguous scleral involvement
- Topical cycloplegic agents and systemic analgesics
- **Other treatment:**
  - tissue adhesive corneal patch grafting • tectonic keratoplasty • conjunctival flap
- Controversy regarding *if* and *when* to use topical steroids
  - When possible, comanage with cornea specialist

Prognosis

- Potentially sight-threatening ocular infection
- May induce rapid destruction of corneal tissue and intraocular spread of infection
- **Severity of corneal infection determined by:**
  - virulence of organism • age • general health and genetic makeup • compliance to treatment • correct choice of antimicrobial therapy

Severe Ulcer

Any of the following:
- central location (visual axis) • epithelial defect >2.0 mm • corneal infiltrate >3.0 mm • rapid progression • involves over one-third of corneal thickness • necrosis of corneal tissue, with impending or overt perforation • scleral involvement • immunosuppressed patient

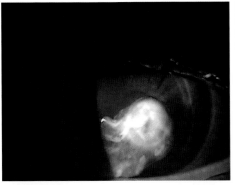

Fig. 5.92 Pseudomonas keratitis: mucopurulent secretion adherent to the ulcer.

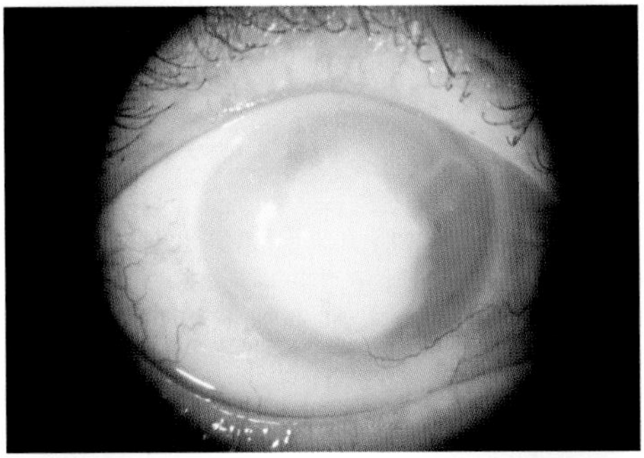

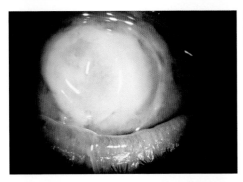

Fig. 5.93 Corneal scarring after infectious keratitis. Penetrating or lamellar keratoplasty is indicated for visual rehabilitation.

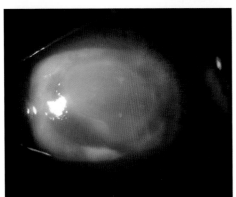

Fig. 5.94 Endophthalmitis secondary to perforated bacterial ulcer.

Fig. 5.95 A large central corneal ulcer delineated by fluorescein. (Courtesy of Bruno F. Fernandes, MD.)

Staphylococcal Marginal Ulcer

Key Facts

- Result of chronic blepharoconjunctivitis
- Hypersensitivity reaction of host's antibody to staphylococcal antigen
- No sex, gender, race, geographic, or age predilection

Clinical Findings

- Inflamed eyelids, lid margin telangiectasia, loss of lashes, collarettes
- Conjunctival papillary and/or follicular reaction
- Superficial punctate keratopathy (most pronounced inferiorly)
- Localized peripheral stromal opacities in oblique meridians, separated from the limbus by a lucid interval
- Peripheral ulceration and/or stromal thinning (may be no associated epithelial defect)
- Peripheral neovascularization
- No alterations seen on anterior chamber

Ancillary Testing

- Corneal scrapings and lid margin samples for microbiologic evaluation
  - Recommend against corneal scraping if epithelium is intact—sometimes to help elucidate bacterial resistance and differential diagnosis to other microorganisms

Differential Diagnosis

- Phlyctenular keratoconjunctivitis (tuberculosis or syphilis)
- Dry eye, peripheral ulcerative keratitis caused by collagen vascular diseases
- Herpetic keratitis
- Peripheral ulcerative keratitis

Treatment

- Topical steroids (fluormetholone 0.1% q.i.d.)
- Topical antibiotics (broad spectrum) when epithelial defects
- **Treat associated blepharitis:**
  - warm compresses and eyelid hygiene (diluted baby shampoo)
  - systemic doxycycline and erythromycin ointment

Prognosis

- Usually non–sight-threatening condition
- Condition may be chronic if blepharitis is not controlled

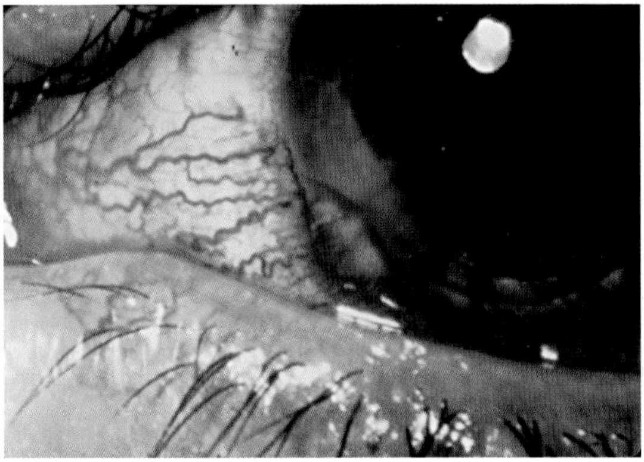

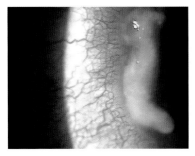

Fig. 5.96 Inflamed eyelid margin, corneal peripheral ulceration, and neovascularization.

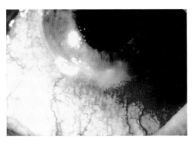

Fig. 5.97 Peripheral stromal opacity with a clear stromal interval separating the lesion from the limbus. Note conjunctival injection.

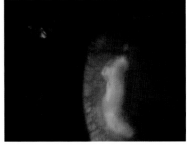

Fig. 5.98 Same patient as in Fig. 5.97, showing fluorescein staining of ulcerated areas.

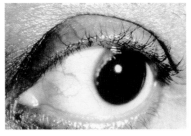

Fig. 5.99 Inferior lesion. Note intense conjunctival inflammation, corneal opacities, and neovascularization.

Fig. 5.100 Superior lesion, with eyelid inflammation, thickened lid margin, and corneal opacities.

Herpes Simplex Virus: Infectious Epithelial Keratopathy

Key Facts

- Incidence of herpes simplex virus (HSV) ocular disease estimated to be 8.4 new cases per 100 000 people per year
- Geographic location, socioeconomic status, and age influence HSV prevalence—it is an increasing health problem
- **Recurrences can be triggered by:**
    - fever • hormonal changes • ultraviolet exposure • psychologic stress • ocular trauma • other infectious diseases • trigeminal nerve manipulation
- Recurrent HSV can present with isolated lid, conjunctival, epithelial, stromal, or intraocular inflammation
- Almost invariably unilateral (bilateral disease in about 10%)
- More common in atopes and immunosuppressed
- Humans are the only reservoir of HSV
- HSV keratitis tends to be more severe in children

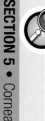

Clinical Findings

- Conjunctival hyperemia and follicular reaction
- **Dendritic ulcers:**
    - branching linear ulcer with terminal bulbs and swollen epithelial borders
    - cornea vesicles, marginal and/or geographic ulcers (scalloped borders) with limbal injection
- Decreased corneal sensation
- Peripheral neovascularization in some cases

Ancillary Testing

- Usually a clinical diagnosis
- Viral culture, PCR, cytologic examination

Differential Diagnosis

- Herpes zoster infection
- *Acanthamoeba* keratitis
- Dendritic keratopathy secondary to long-term topical trifluridine
- Healing corneal abrasion

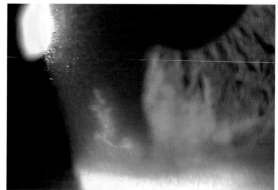

Fig. 5.101 Peripheral dendritic lesion with surrounding edema.

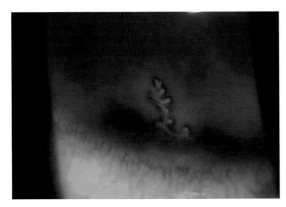

Fig. 5.102 Same patient as in Fig. 5.97: fluorescein staining epithelial defect. Note terminal bulbs.

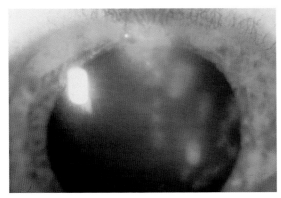

Fig. 5.103 Herpetic epithelial infection with associated limbitis. Note numerous lesions with surrounding edema.

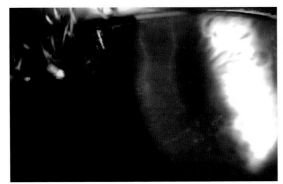

Fig. 5.104 Herpetic neuritis: note thick and pronounced corneal nerves.

Treatment

- Mechanical debridement of ulcers
- Topical trifluridine 1% drops every 2 h for 10–14 days
- Vidarabine 3% ointment five times a day (particularly helpful in children) for 10–14 days
- Topical acyclovir ointment five times daily (not available in the USA) for 10–14 days
- Oral acyclovir is effective in adults and children
- Topical cycloplegics
- Steroids not recommended unless presents with severe immune stromal inflammation
- **Other treatment:**
    - systemic doxycycline • tarsorrhaphy • conjunctival flaps • tissue adhesives
        - lamellar or penetrating keratoplasty

Prognosis

- >90% of patients maintain good visual acuity despite prolonged disease
- Stromal scarring can cause thinning and decreased vision
- Oral acyclovir is effective in decreasing the incidence of recurrent HSV epithelial and stromal disease
- Topical steroids do not significantly increase risk of recurrent epithelial disease
- HIV-positive patients have the same clinical course but increased risk of recurrence
- Vaccine initiatives have not yet been fruitful

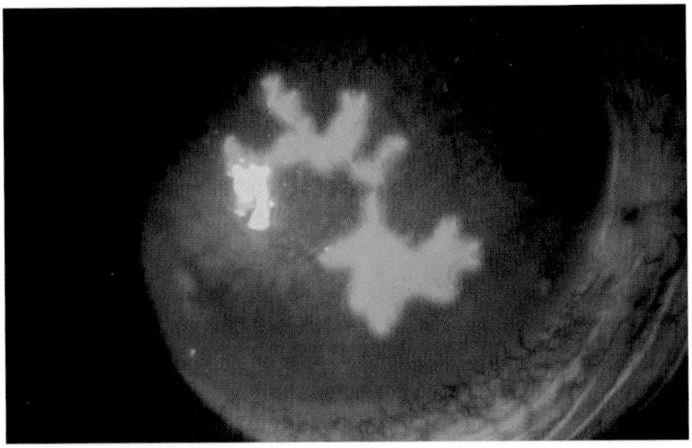

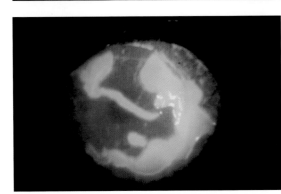

Fig. 5.105 Central dendritic herpetic lesion stained with fluorescein.

Fig. 5.106 Corneal geographic ulcer: associated corneal hypesthesia.

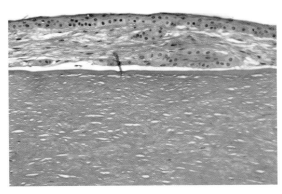

Fig. 5.107 Corneal scar secondary to herpes simplex keratitis. Multiple layers of epithelium and aberrant basement membrane deposition. Periodic acid Schiff, ×100. (Courtesy of Bruno F. Fernandes, MD, and Miguel N. Burnier Jr., MD, PhD.)

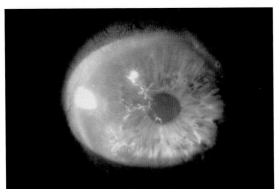

Fig. 5.108 Another example of a typical central corneal dendritic lesion.

Herpes Simplex Virus: Immune Stromal Keratitis

Key Facts

- Antigen–antibody complement–mediated, possibly due to retained viral antigen within stroma
- About 20–25% of patients with herpetic eye disease develop stromal keratitis
- Incidence of herpes simplex virus (HSV) ocular disease is estimated to be 8.4 new cases per 100 000 people per year
- Recurrent HSV can present with isolated lid, conjunctival, epithelial, stromal, or intraocular inflammation
- Almost invariably unilateral (bilateral disease in about 10%)
- More common in atopes and immunosuppressed
- HSV keratitis tends to be more severe in children

Clinical Findings

- Conjunctival hyperemia, ciliary flush, anterior chamber reaction
- Overlying epithelium is almost always intact (except when combined with epithelial disease)
- Stromal infiltration, punctate stromal opacities
- Neovascularization at any level of the cornea, ghost vessels
- Immune ring, edema, limbitis
- Thinning, scarring, lipid deposition

Ancillary Testing

- Usually clinical diagnosis

Differential Diagnosis

- Syphilitic or tuberculosis interstitial keratitis
- Herpes zoster keratitis

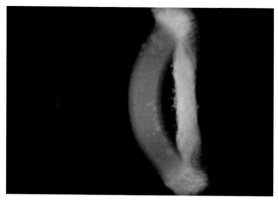

Fig. 5.109 Conjunctival injection and corneal stromal opacities with surrounding edema.

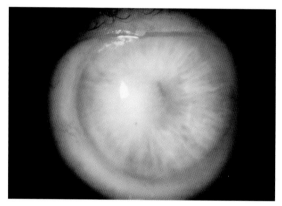

Fig. 5.110 Herpetic stromal keratitis sequelae: corneal neovascularization and scarring.

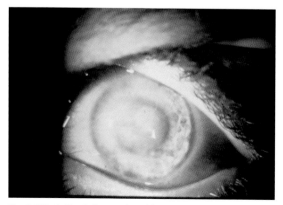

Fig. 5.111 Active inflammation. Note lipid deposition and corneal inflammatory edema.

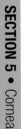

Treatment

- Topical (sometimes also systemic) steroids (prednisolone acetate 1% every 2 h, with slow tapering)
- Topical cycloplegics
- Oral acyclovir is not effective in controlling active stromal keratitis but should be used (400 mg twice daily) as prophylaxis during steroid therapy
- **Other treatment:**
  - systemic doxycycline • tarsorrhaphy • conjunctival flaps • tissue adhesives
    - lamellar or penetrating keratoplasty

Prognosis

- **May lead to:**
  - stromal thinning • scarring • neovascularization • lipid deposition • severe loss of vision
- Topical steroids reduce persistence and progression of stromal inflammation
- Patients submitted to penetrating keratoplasty are at high risk of developing recurrence of active infection in the graft
- Oral acyclovir is effective in decreasing the incidence of recurrent HSV ocular disease, particularly stromal with a history of recurrence
- HIV-positive patients have the same clinical course but increased risk of recurrence
- Vaccine initiatives have not yet been fruitful

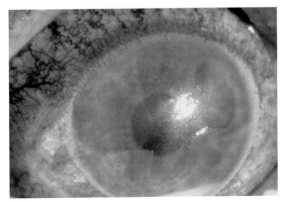

Fig. 5.112 Acute herpetic associated iritis and immune stromal keratitis. Conjunctival injection and hypopyon are seen.

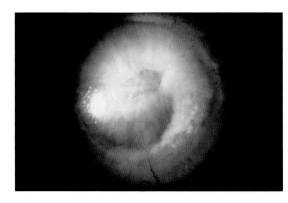

Fig. 5.113 Stromal keratitis with neovascularization.

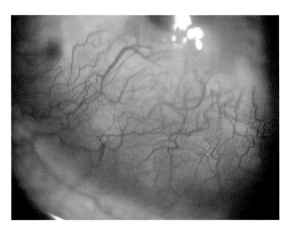

Fig. 5.114 Superficial neovascular pannus in the inferior cornea. (Courtesy of Bruno F. Fernandes, MD.)

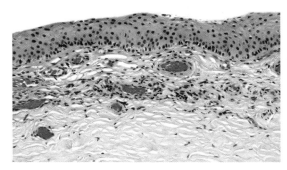

Fig. 5.115 Superficial corneal neovascularization and subepithelial fibrosis. The epithelium is acanthotic, and Bowman's layer is absent. Hematoxylin and eosin, ×100. (Courtesy of Bruno F. Fernandes, MD, and Miguel N. Burnier Jr., MD, PhD).

Herpes Simplex Viral Disciform Endotheliitis

Key Facts

- Most common cause of central non-bacterial keratitis
- **Associated with:**
  - sun exposure • fever • stress • menses • trauma • illness
    - immunosuppression
- High incidence of recurrence
- May be self-limited (2–6 months)

Clinical Findings

- Focal disc-like stromal edema
- Corneal Descemet's folds
- Keratic precipitates only within areas of edema
- Scarring if previous episodes
- Increased IOP if concomitant trabeculitis
- Anterior chamber cells and flare less than expected from number of keratic precipitates

Ancillary Testing

- Corneal pachymetry
- Photographic documentation

Differential Diagnosis

- Corneal trauma
- Bullous keratopathy
- Endothelial dysfunction

Treatment

- **Topical steroid:** prednisolone acetate 1% q.h., depending on severity
- Cycloplegic agent
- Topical antiviral if epithelium involved
- Oral suppressive therapy with acyclovir 400 mg p.o. b.i.d.
- Topical beta blocker or prostaglandin inhibitor to control IOP

Prognosis

- Recurrence rate 25% during first year, 50% during second year
- Long-term suppressive therapy with acyclovir 400 mg p.o. b.i.d. for 1 year with 6-month follow-up reduces incidence of recurrent keratitis by almost 50% (Herpetic Eye Disease Study conclusion)

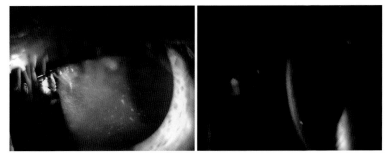

Fig. 5.116 Localized corneal edema with posterior keratic precipitates and pigments.

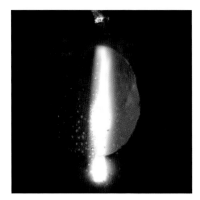

Fig. 5.117 Retroillumination of the same patient as in Fig. 5.116. Note segmental iris atrophy.

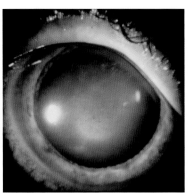

Fig. 5.118 Disciform keratitis: localized endothelial inflammation with corresponding stromal edema.

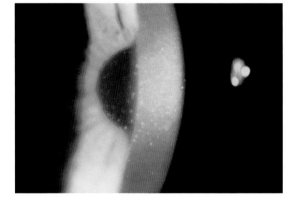

Fig. 5.119 Stromal edema, keratic precipitates, endothelial pigment, and anterior chamber reaction.

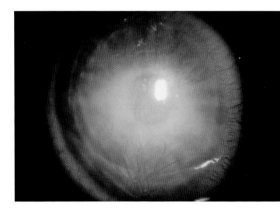

Fig. 5.120 Another example of herpetic endothelial inflammation and central corneal edema.

Varicella-zoster Virus

Key Facts

- Varicella-zoster virus is a member of the Herpesviridae family, which infects >95% of the adult US population
- No race, gender, geographic, or seasonal preference
- Increased risk for developing disease in patients with altered cell-mediated immunity

Clinical Findings

- Vesicular eyelid lesions or conjunctivitis
- Superficial punctate keratopathy
- Raised, plaque-like dendritic keratopathy that is different from herpes simplex virus (HSV) dendritic keratitis (which is a true ulcer)
- Nummular sub-Bowman's layer infiltrates
- Decreased corneal sensation, necrotizing corneal inflammation (with or without corneal melting)
- Stromal neovascularization, disciform keratitis, limbitis
- Increased IOP, hyphema, iridocyclitis, cataract
- Extraocular muscle paresis, episcleritis, scleritis
- Retinitis, choroiditis, optic neuritis

Ancillary Testing

- Usually a clinical diagnosis
- Tzanck smear to confirm multinucleated giant cells, immunofluorescent and immunoenzyme stains
- PCR, culture of vesicular fluid, serologic tests

Differential Diagnosis

- HSV keratitis
- Zoster dendrites lack the characteristic terminal bulbs of HSV dendrites and are often more linear and less branched
- *Acanthamoeba* keratitis
- Impetigo

Treatment

- Oral acyclovir (800 mg five times daily), famciclovir (125 mg four times daily), or valaciclovir (1000 mg three times daily) for 7–19 days
- Immunocompromised patients require intravenous medication (acyclovir 15–20 mg/kg per day) for ≥5 days
- Surgical therapy include tarsorrhaphy, corneal grafts, and conjunctival flaps

Prognosis

- Can lead to blindness and long-term ocular morbidity
- Hutchinson sign (presence of vesicles at side of tip of nose) is a poor prognostic indicator
- Penetrating keratoplasty has showed poor results in numerous studies and requires concomitant tarsorrhaphy in most cases

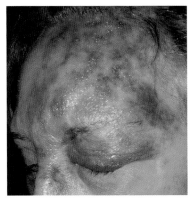

Fig. 5.121 Facial zoster infection: hemifacial swelling, hyperemia, and typical skin lesions.

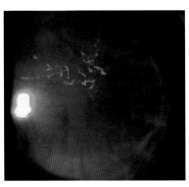

Fig. 5.122 Zoster dendritiform epithelial defects stained with fluorescein. Note linear aspect and absence of terminal bulbs.

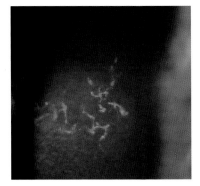

Fig. 5.123 Same patient as in Fig. 5.122, image in detail.

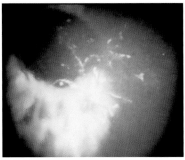

Fig. 5.124 Another example of epithelial keratitis with typical zoster dendritiform lesions.

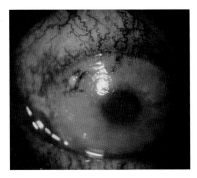

Fig. 5.125 Acute severe zoster sclerokeratouveitis. Diffuse and severe inflammation.

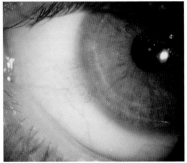

Fig. 5.126 Zoster localized limbitis.

Fungal Keratitis

Key Facts

- Important cause of visual loss in developing countries
- Incidence, risk factors, and causative agent vary among different geographic regions
- **Two classic basic forms described:**
  1. Caused by filamentous fungi (especially *Fusarium* and *Aspergillus*)
     - Trauma is the key predisposing factor, more common in healthy young males
  2. Caused by yeast-like and related fungi (particularly *Candida*)
     - Usually concomitant pre-existing ocular and/or systemic disease

Clinical Findings

- Firm elevated areas, hyphate lines extending into unaffected cornea
- Multifocal granular (or feathery) grey-white satellite stromal infiltrates
- Immune ring or nummular midstromal infiltrates
- Descemet's folds, iritis, endothelial plaque, hypopyon

Ancillary Testing

- Microbiologic investigation (material obtained by corneal scraping or biopsy)
  - Microscopy: potassium hydroxide 10%, gram, Giemsa, periodic acid Schiff, calcofluor white
  - Culture (may require incubation for ≤4–6 weeks): blood agar, brain–heart infusion agar, Sabouraud agar, thioglycolate broth

Differential Diagnosis

- Bacterial keratitis
- Herpetic keratitis

Treatment

- **First-line therapy for superficial keratitis (continued for ≥6 weeks):**
  - topical natamycin 5% or amphotericin B 0.15% (hourly around the clock for several days)
  - deep lesions necessitate subconjunctival and/or systemic therapy as well (miconazole, ketoconazole, itraconazole, fluconazole)
- **Surgical treatment includes:**
  - debridement of infected or necrotic tissue • conjunctival flaps • tissue adhesives • penetrating keratoplasty
- Cycloplegics

Prognosis

- Can lead to blindness in a few weeks depending on interplay of agent, host, and predisposing factors
- Slow response to treatment can be expected, corticosteroids can lead to worsening
- 15–27% of patients require surgical intervention because of failure of medical therapy

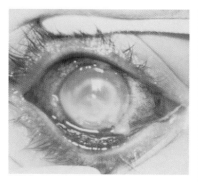

Fig. 5.127 *Aspergillus* keratitis: severe ocular inflammation, corneal immune ring, and hypopyon.

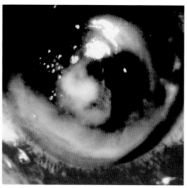

Fig. 5.128 Grey-white elevated corneal lesion with undistinct margins and satellite infiltrates.

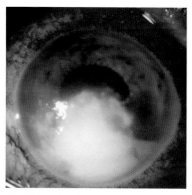

Fig. 5.129 *Fusarium solani* keratitis: extensive lesion with associated hypopion. (Courtesy of the External Eye Disease and Cornea Section, Federal University of Sao Paulo, Brazil.)

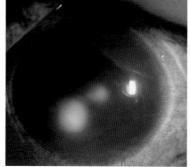

Fig. 5.130 *Candida* keratitis in a diabetic patient. (Courtesy of the External Eye Disease and Cornea Section, Federal University of Sao Paulo, Brazil.)

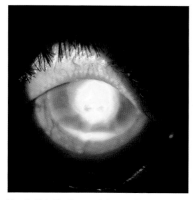

Fig. 5.131 Perforated Aspergillus keratitis. Shallow anterior chamber and hypopion.

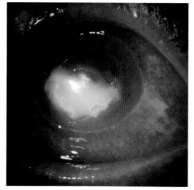

Fig. 5.132 *Fusarium* keratitis: indistinct feathered edges and diffuse stromal invasion. (Courtesy of the External Eye Disease and Cornea Section, Federal University of Sao Paulo, Brazil.)

Atypical Bacteria

Key Facts

- Opportunistic pathogens—requires alteration in normal environment to cause infection
- Non-tuberculous or atypical mycobacteria are the most common etiologic factors in post-LASIK infections
- Clusters or outbreaks in laser vision correction centers around the world have been described
- **Mycobacterium species found in:**
  - water • milk • soil • animals • scrub sinks • skin • sputum • the environment
- Rod-shaped, non-motile, non–spore-forming aerobic bacteria referred to as acid-fast bacilli
- Indolent course, with delayed onset of symptoms (usually 1–3 weeks) after risk event (e.g. trauma or surgery)

Clinical Findings

- Focal, round, or dot-like whitish infiltrates • Dust-like ring of tiny white opacities surrounding a major larger infiltrate • Cracked windshield appearance • Satellite lesions • Flap necrosis (if after LASIK)

Ancillary Testing

- **Microbiologic evaluation (corneal scraping or biopsy):**
  - smears (gram, Giemsa, Ziehl–Neelsen, fluorochrome stains)
  - culture (blood and chocolate agar, thioglycolate broth, Lowenstein–Jensen media)
  - antimicrobial susceptibility testing
- PCR

Differential Diagnosis

- Bacterial (especially *Nocardia* and *Corynebacterium*) or fungal keratitis • Infectious crystalline keratopathy • Diffuse lamellar keratitis

Treatment

- **Topical antibiotics:**
  - tobramycin 14 mg/mL • amikacin 50 mg/mL • clarithromycin 10 mg/mL • ofloxacin 3 mg/mL • azithromycin 2 mg/mL • fluoroquinolones (gatifloxacin 0.3% or moxifloxacin 0.5%)
- Systemic clarithromycin (500 mg twice a day)
- Surgical debridement or therapeutic lamellar keratectomy (sometimes flap removal is necessary)
- Topical cycloplegics
- Steroids are contraindicated

Prognosis

- Location in the flap interface after LASIK can make it more difficult to obtain samples for microbiologic evaluation and prevent adequate concentration of antibiotics
- Sight-threatening infection
- Early diagnosis and institution of appropriate treatment are crucial to satisfactory outcome
- Long-term treatment—patient compliance is crucial

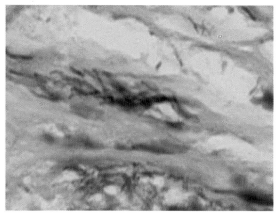

Fig. 5.133 Corneal biopsy showing the mycobacterium. (Courtesy of Filipe A. Gusmao, MD.)

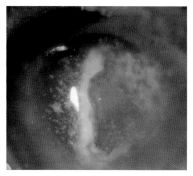

Fig. 5.134 Mycobacteria keratitis (acute phase): cornel infiltrates with multiple dots and crystalline keratopathy. (Courtesy of Filipe A. Gusmao, MD.)

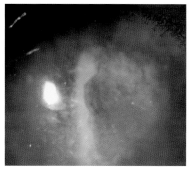

Fig. 5.135 Irregular infiltrate, indistinct margins, and satellite lesions. (Courtesy of Filipe A. Gusmao, MD.)

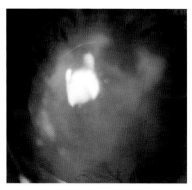

Fig. 5.136 Mycobacteria keratitis: healing phase. (Courtesy of Filipe A. Gusmao, MD.)

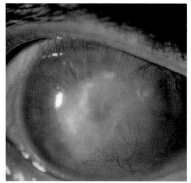

Fig. 5.137 Mycobacteria keratitis: healing phase. (Courtesy of Filipe A. Gusmao, MD.)

Acanthamoeba Keratitis

Key Facts

- Contact lens wear is strongest risk factor, with soft hydrogel lenses responsible for most cases
- Incidence of one case per 30 000 contact lens wearers per year
- **Acanthamoeba can be isolated from about 15% of contact lens storage cases and is also found in:**
  - chlorinated swimming pools • showers • jacuzzis • fountains • sandy beaches • seawater • ocean sediment • sewage outfalls
- Use of tap water for contact lens hygiene is strongly related to infection (source of *Acanthamoeba*)
- Only four *Acanthamoeba* genotypes (T3, T4, T6, and T11) have been associated with keratitis
- The organism is characterized by a life cycle of feeding and replicating trophozoite and dormant cyst stages
- Characteristic symptom is a disproportionately severe ocular pain not commensurate with clinical findings

Clinical Findings

- Paracentral ring-like stromal infiltrate, epithelial haze • Epithelial defects and stromal nummular infiltrates • Dendritiform ulcers, epithelial irregularities and erosions • Limbitis or radial keratoneuritis • Diffuse or nodular scleritis, anterior chamber reaction

Ancillary Testing

- Corneal scrapings and biopsy to microbiologic evaluation
  - direct microscopy (calcofluor white, gram, Giemsa, acridine orange)
  - culture (*Escherichia coli* plated on non-nutrient agar 1.5%)
- Confocal microscopy or PCR

Differential Diagnosis

- Herpetic keratitis • Bacterial or fungal keratitis

Treatment

- Epithelial debridement improves penetration of drugs into cornea and should be done in early phases • Propamidine isethionate 0.1% (Brolene) • Polyhexamethylene biguanide 0.02% • Topical chlorhexidine 0.02% • Neomycin–polymyxin B–gramicidin • Systemic ketoconazole (200–600 mg/day) • Penetrating keratoplasty when impending perforation • Topical cycloplegics and non-steroidal anti-inflammatory drugs • Steroids have a deleterious effect and are contraindicated

Prognosis

- Vision-threatening disease—permanent visual loss in >30% of patients and enucleation in recalcitrant cases
- The resistance of *Acanthamoeba* cysts to most antimicrobial agents makes it one of the most difficult ocular infections to treat, with a mean treatment period of >5 months and surgical interventions in ≤50% of cases
- Patient's compliance to treatment is difficult but critical
- Graft recurrence of the infection is common, so penetrant keratoplasty should be delayed until the disease is under control

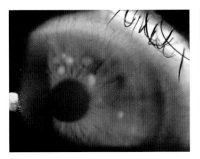

Fig. 5.138 *Acanthamoeba* infection in a soft contact lens wearer. Nummular lesions with little conjunctival injection.

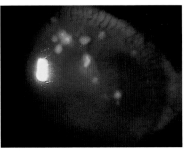

Fig. 5.139 Same patient as in Fig. 5.138: fluorescein staining due to epithelial defect.

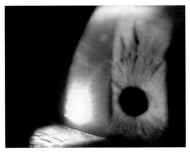

Fig. 5.140 Typical sign: radial neuritis. A pain disproportional to the extent of corneal inflammation is usually found in these patients.

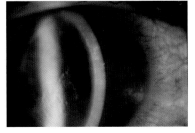

Fig. 5.141 Dendritiform epithelial lesions. Herpetic keratitis is one differential diagnosis. (Courtesy of Denise de Freitas, MD.)

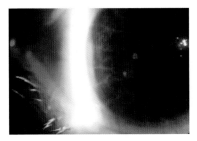

Fig. 5.142 Another example of evident corneal nerve inflammation in acanthamoebic keratitis. (Courtesy of Denise de Freitas, MD.)

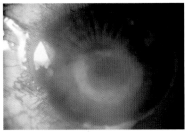

Fig. 5.143 Immune ring in amoebic keratitis, with surrounding edema. Pronounced ciliary injection. (Courtesy of Denise de Freitas, MD.)

Corneal Abrasion

Key Facts

- One of the most common eye injuries, with an estimated incidence of 789 in 100 000
- Most commonly seen after a tangential impact from a foreign body, radiation, heat and chemical trauma
- Keep in mind that occult ocular injuries may be present

Clinical Findings

- **Topical anesthetic facilitates the examination, which shows:**
  - conjunctival hyperemia
  - loss of corneal luster
  - epithelial defect with surrounding loose epithelium
  - a granular anterior stromal infiltrate underlying the defect (if the examination is delayed)
  - normal anterior chamber

Ancillary Testing

- Clinical diagnosis (history and slit-lamp examination with fluorescein staining)

Differential Diagnosis

- Factitious keratoconjunctivitis
- Source of injury (mechanical, chemical, thermal)

Treatment

- Topical cycloplegic
- Topical broad-spectrum antibiotic (e.g. fluoroquinolone or aminoglycoside)
- Bandage contact lens (preferable), taping of lids, or application of a pressure patch

Prognosis

- Most cases have a favorable outcome, with complete healing in 1–2 days
- Bowman's membrane lesion leads to scarring
- Increased risk for bacterial infection while epithelial defect exists—close follow-up is warranted

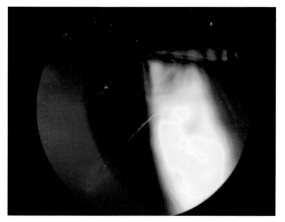

Fig. 5.144 Traumatic corneal lesion (piece of paper). This patient had epithelial erosion 2 weeks after total wound healing.

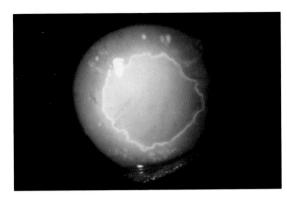

Fig. 5.145 Central epithelial defect due to alkali burn: clear borders with well-defined margins.

Fig. 5.146 Intrastromal foreign body.

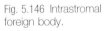

Fig. 5.147 Corneal lesion with positive Seidel testing. Leakage can be seen in the inferior aspect.

Recurrent Erosion Secondary to Trauma

Key Facts

- Can be secondary to trivial trauma (e.g. from a fingernail, the edge of paper, or a leaf of a tree)
- Characterized by repeated episodes of pain, photophobia, watering, redness, and tearing, especially on awakening
- Related to poor adhesion of corneal epithelium to underlying stroma
- Incidence is about 1 in 150 cases following traumatic corneal abrasion

Clinical Findings

- Most commonly occurring within lower half of cornea
- Corneal epithelial defects
- Loosely adherent and elevated epithelium
- Epithelial microcysts
- Stromal infiltrates and/or opacities

Ancillary Testing

- Clinical diagnosis (history and slit-lamp examination)

Differential Diagnosis

- Factitious keratoconjunctivitis
- Exposure keratitis or neurotrophic keratopathy
- Herpetic keratitis
- Foreign bodies under tarsal plate

Treatment

- **Clinical:**
  - patching, cycloplegia, topical lubrication and antibiotics, bandage contact lens
  - autologous serum, oral doxycycline, botulinum toxin–induced ptosis
- **Surgical:**
  - diamond burr polishing of Bowman's membrane
  - anterior stromal puncture
  - phototherapeutic keratectomy

Prognosis

- May rarely lead to visual disability
- Most cases respond well to conservative (clinical) treatment
- Corneal infiltrates and infectious keratitis may develop at site of corneal erosions
- Long-term use of contact lenses may predispose to bacterial keratitis, vascularization, and scarring

Factitious Keratoconjunctivitis

Key Facts

- Psychopathologic condition in which symptoms or physical findings are intentionally produced in order to assume the sick role
  - Self-induced or accidental trauma is emphatically denied
- Rare and difficult to diagnose condition
- Can result from mechanical or chemical trauma
- Most common in military personnel and medical field employees
- A confession as to self-inflicting an artificial ocular disease is attained in only few patients

Clinical Findings

- **Chronic (usually >3 weeks) conjunctivitis with peculiar characteristics:**
  - purulent discharge • nearly always localized inferiorly (with quiet superior bulbar conjunctiva) • severe hyperemia and mild chemosis • punctate keratopathy, coarse focal keratopathy, persistent epithelial defect
- Filamentary keratopathy or pseudodendrites

Ancillary Testing

- Clinical diagnosis (history and slit-lamp examination)

Differential Diagnosis

- Toxic keratoconjunctivitis, allergic diseases, blepharitis, dry eye
- Munchausen syndrome by proxy, malingering, neurologic disorders
- Mucus fishing syndrome, congenital or acquired corneal anesthesia
- Topical anesthetic abuse

Treatment

- **Depends on extent and presentation of each case:**
  - patching, bandage contact lens, topical antibiotics, and preservative-free artificial tears
  - Sometimes requires hospitalization
- Psychiatric evaluation is typically indicated

Prognosis

- Visual outcome depends on extent of self-inflicted damage
- Dramatic improvement of clinical findings is found when patient is placed under 24-h observation

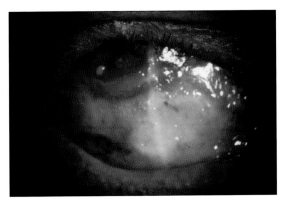

Fig. 5.148 Inferior conjunctival ulceration, with associated corneal epithelial defect and severe hyperemia. (Courtesy of Ivan Schwab, MD.)

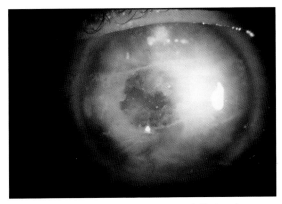

Fig. 5.149 Severe end stage disease: calcific band keratopathy due to chronic inflammation. (Courtesy of Ivan Schwab, MD.)

Chemical and Thermal Injuries

Key Facts

- Incidence is about 7.7–18% of all ocular trauma
- Alkali (most commonly ammonia) injuries are more frequent than acid (most commonly sulfuric acid) injuries
- Higher incidence among males at younger ages (16–30 years)
- **Most common sites of exposure:**
  - at home • at work • in association with violence

Clinical Findings

- **Acute phase:**
  - conjunctival hyperemia and chemosis
  - epithelial defects, coagulation, and devitalization of corneal epithelium
  - corneal edema and stromal cloudiness
  - limbal ischemia and thrombosed conjunctival blood vessels
  - mydriasis, anterior chamber reaction, cataract

Ancillary Testing

- Clinical diagnosis (history and slit-lamp examination)

Differential Diagnosis

- Factitious keratoconjunctivitis
- Recurrent erosion syndrome
- Mechanical traumatic corneal abrasion

Treatment

- **Abundant ocular irrigation (after topical anesthetic drops), preferably with sterile solutions (e.g. lactated Ringer solution and balanced saline solution), then:**
  - topical antibiotics, preservative-free artificial tears, patching and bandage contact lens in mild cases
  - add intensive steroid therapy, oral doxycycline, surgical debridement of necrotic tissue in moderate to severe cases
  - in very severe cases, consider amniotic membrane transplantation, tenoplasty, limbal stem cell transplantation (once acute inflammation has resolved), penetrating keratoplasty, keratoprosthesis

Prognosis

- Most injuries do not cause lasting damage but others can result in permanent blindness
- Close and long-term follow-up is crucial, and visual rehabilitation is sometimes a slow and challenging process
- In general, alkalis penetrate more rapidly and cause more damage than acids
  - Irreversible damage occurs at pH >11.5
- **The time between lesion and ocular irrigation has the greatest influence on prognosis, but also important are:**
  - severity of injury (mostly extent of limbal ischemia) • duration of exposure
    - type of chemical • volume • concentration (pH)

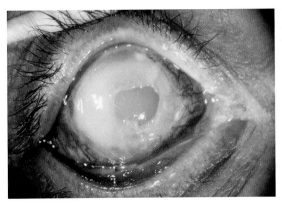

Fig. 5.150 Severe alkali burn: diffuse conjunctival hyperemia, limbal ischemia, epithelial defect, and corneal loss of luster.

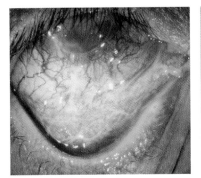

Fig. 5.151 Conjunctival and limbal lesion.

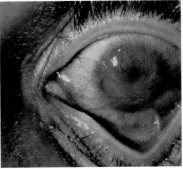

Fig. 5.152 Alkali burn sequela: corneal neovascularization and scarring, with loss of vision.

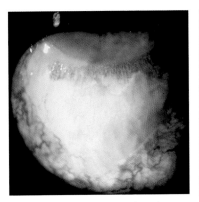

Fig. 5.153 Conjunctival staining after chemical burn.

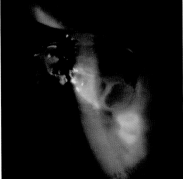

Fig. 5.154 Corneal ulcer secondary to thermal injury.

Section 6
Iris and Ciliary Body

Idiopathic Iritis

Key Facts

- Occurs in any age, no sex predilection
- No systemic disease associated, do not have the HLA-B27 haplotype
- Etiologic factor unknown
- Non-granulomatous inflammation more common than granulomatous
- Most common complaints are redness, pain, and photophobia

Clinical Findings

- Conjunctival injection, ciliary flush
- Presence of cells and flare in anterior chamber
- Keratic precipitates
- Pupillary miosis, dilated iris vessels
- Posterior synechiae and hypopyon are rare findings but can occur

Ancillary Testing

- Assess complete medical history and thorough examination
- **Rule out:**
  - Ocular diseases (herpes, Fuchs heterochromic iridocyclitis, and others)
  - Syphilis (VDRL test, fluorescent treponemal antibody absorption test)
  - Connective tissue disease (complete blood cell count, urinalysis)
  - Tuberculosis and/or sarcoidosis (purified protein derivative, chest x-ray, calcium tests, serum angiotensin-converting enzyme level)

Differential Diagnosis

- Masquerade syndromes (malignancies, including leukemia and lymphoma)
- Intraocular foreign bodies
- Infectious cause (e.g. herpetic uveitis)
- Pigment dispersion syndrome
- Systemic diseases with ocular manifestations

Treatment

- Topical corticosteroids (prednisolone acetate 1%)
- Topical cycloplegic and mydriatic agents
- Topical hypotensive agents when high IOP (avoid use of pilocarpine and prostaglandin agonists)

Prognosis

- Patients with anterior uveitis can develop posterior segment disease
- Secondary glaucoma and cataract can develop due to chronic treatment with steroids
- Recurrent episodes of ocular inflammation can occur

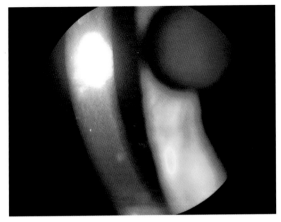

Fig. 6.1 Small keratic precipitates during acute
inflammation, composed of neutrophils and lymphocytes.

Sarcoidosis

Key Facts

- Multisystem immunologic granulomatous disease can affect almost every organ (most commonly the lungs, thoracic lymph nodes, and skin, whereas the adrenal glands are consistently spared by the disease), characterized by formation of non-caseating epithelioid cell granulomas
- Ocular manifestations occur in 25–50% of patients and are more common in darkly pigmented people with chronic disease
- Usually bilateral (about 90%) but may be unilateral or asymmetric

Clinical Findings

- **Anterior granulomatous uveitis is the most common ocular manifestation (53–60% of patients):**
  - mutton fat keratic precipitates
  - iris nodules (Koeppe and Busacca)
  - anterior chamber inflammation
  - posterior synechiae
- Conjunctival granulomas (7–17% of patients with ocular involvement)
- Secondary cataract (8–17% of patients) and glaucoma (11–23% of patients)
- Episcleritis, scleritis
- Vitritis, snowballs, macular edema, perivenous sheathing, optic disk swelling, retinal neovascularization

Ancillary Testing

- Confirm diagnosis (purified protein derivative, angiotensin-converting enzyme level, chest radiography)—refer to a clinician
- Conjunctival and/or nodular skin lesion biopsy (look for non-caseating granuloma)
- B scan to assess posterior segment or optical coherence tomography to evaluate macular edema
- Fluorescein angiography

Differential Diagnosis

- Tuberculosis
- Vogt–Koyanagi–Harada disease • Iris malignancies • Coats disease
  - Rheumatoid arthritis

Treatment

- The mainstay of therapy for both systemic and ocular disease is corticosteroids
- Sometimes ocular inflammation requires periocular injections and/or oral steroids
- Methotrexate, cyclosporine, and other systemic immunosuppressive agents also have therapeutic effects
- Topical cycloplegic and mydriatic agents
- IOP control, cataract and/or vitreoretinal surgery when indicated

Prognosis

- Sight-threatening condition—about 15% of eyes show severe visual loss
- Treatment of several ocular complications (band keratopathy, cataract, glaucoma, chronic macular edema, and others) is often challenging
- Some patients show complete remission within several years, while some show persistent inflammation

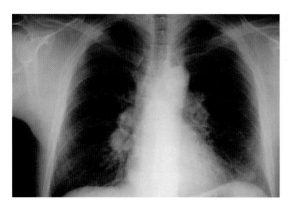

Fig. 6.2 Chest x-ray in a patient with sarcoidosis: hilar adenopathy.

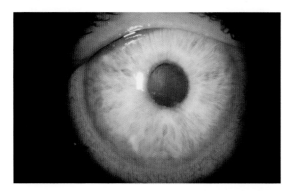

Fig. 6.3 Sarcoid conjunctival granuloma.

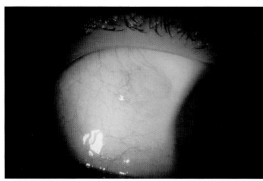

Fig. 6.4 Anterior uveitis: iris nodules (both Koeppe and Busacca).

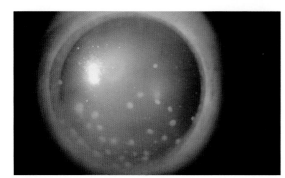

Fig. 6.5 Mutton fat keratic precipitates in a patient with granulomatous anterior chamber inflammation due to sarcoidosis.

Fuchs Heterochromatic Iridocyclitis

Key Facts

- Classic hallmark is iris heterochromia (sometimes difficult to recognize)
- 7–15% of patients have bilateral involvement
- Typically affects young patients and causes mild blurred vision
- Pain and redness are rare
- Cataract is commonly associated

Clinical Findings

- Heterochromia and/or blurring of the iris stroma with loss of detail and density of iris surface
- Small stellate keratic precipitates with fine filaments uniformly scattered over endothelium
- Mild anterior chamber reaction
- Cataract, high IOP
- Abnormal vessels bridging anterior chamber (neovascularization is rare)
- Mild vitritis and cystoid macular edema can rarely occur

Ancillary Testing

- B scan to evaluate posterior segment when advanced cataract
- Specular microscopy can detail keratic precipitates

Differential Diagnosis

- Malignant melanoma of the iris
- Horner syndrome, Posner–Schlossmann syndrome
- Neovascular glaucoma, chronic anterior uveitis with iris atrophy (e.g. herpes zoster)

Treatment

- **Topical steroids:** controversial—long-term use often unnecessary
- Topical IOP-lowering medications, may need surgery
- Cataract extraction

Prognosis

- Generally a chronic disease
- Cataract surgery has increased risk of hyphema but great visual prognosis
- Glaucoma associated with the disease may be difficult to control and may need tube shunt devices

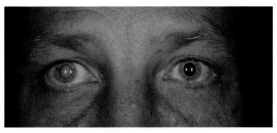

Fig. 6.6 Fine stromal defects in the iris of the affected eye. This image gives almost all the findings, although the heterchromia is subtle. (Courtesy of Ivan Schwab, MD.)

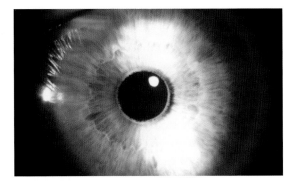

Fig. 6.7 Diffuse stromal iris atrophy with loss of the yellowish points on the collarette—a real marker for Fuchs. (Courtesy of Ivan Schwab, MD.)

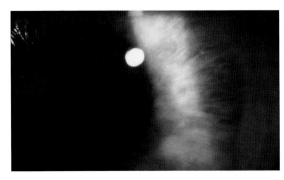

Fig. 6.8 Iris stromal atrophy with the vessels showing through. (Courtesy of Ivan Schwab, MD.)

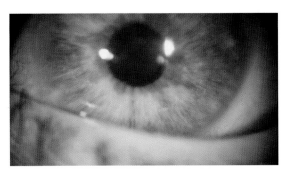

Fig. 6.9 Atrophy, pale iris, and stromal radial vessels. (Courtesy of Ivan Schwab, MD.)

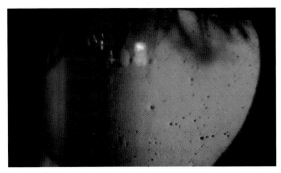

Fig. 6.10 Stellate keratic precipitates in real life are virtually pathognomonic (only herpes simplex virus will show similar morphology). Very fine spikes and diffuse distribution. (Courtesy of Ivan Schwab, MD.)

Juvenile Idiopathic Arthritis

Key Facts

- Formerly known as juvenile rheumatoid arthritis
- Diagnosis of juvenile idiopathic arthritis (JIA) is usually made by the presence of arthritis in a child (<16 years old) with negative rheumatoid factor test and no other cause for joint disease
- Patients with pauciarticular (one to four joints affected) form of JIA have a much higher risk for developing uveitis, especially antinuclear antibody–positive girls
- Usually asymptomatic and insidious with chronic inflammation, predominantly involves iris and ciliary body
- May present as an acute (usually in boys) or chronic indolent (usually in girls) anterior chamber disease

Clinical Findings

- Ciliary flush, conjunctival injection
- Keratic precipitates (mainly in inferior half of corneal endothelium), band keratopathy
- Non-granulomatous anterior chamber inflammation (cells and flare)
- Posterior synechiae with secondary corectopia
- Cataract, high or low IOP
- Vitritis, macular edema

Ancillary Testing

- Rule out sarcoidosis (serum calcium level, chest radiography, serum angiotensin-converting enzyme level)
- B scan to evaluate posterior segment when posterior synechiae

Differential Diagnosis

- Ocular sarcoidosis, juvenile Reiter syndrome, ankylosing spondylitis
- Lyme disease, ocular herpetic disease, Kawasaki disease
- Trauma, inflammatory bowel disease–associated anterior uveitis

Treatment

- Topical steroids are the mainstay of uveitis therapy
- In some cases, periocular injections of depot steroid preparations are needed
- Topical cycloplegic and mydriatic agents
- Topical non-steroidal anti-inflammatory drugs may allow reduction in steroid use
- Cataract surgery to prevent amblyopia (only when inflammation is under control for at least 3 months, IOL implantation is not indicated, consider removal of posterior capsule and anterior vitrectomy)
- Glaucoma control with topical medications and sometimes surgery (consider filtering devices)
- Band keratopathy can be treated with chemical chelation or phototherapeutic keratectomy with the excimer laser

Prognosis

- Sight-threatening condition—evaluation should be made every 3–4 months
- Severity of uveitis is unrelated to severity of underlying joint disease
- **Ocular complications include:**
  - cataract • glaucoma • cystoid macular edema • band keratopathy
    - amblyopia

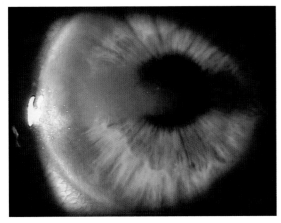

Fig. 6.11 Band keratopathy in a patient with juvenile idiopathic arthritis and chronic anterior uveitis.